SCHOOL

WEST

D0537561

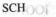

Physics for Medical Imaging

Physics for Medical Imaging

RF Farr MA
Lately Chief Physicist, United Birmingham Hospitals
Senior Clinical Lecturer, University of Birmingham
Medical School, UK

and

PJ Allisy-Roberts PhD MSRP FIPSM
Previously Director of Medical Physics, Southampton University Hospitals,
Physicist (Ionizing radiation dosimetry) Bureau International des Poids et
Mesures, Sèvres, France

With a contribution from **J Weir**, MBBS DMRD FRCP(ed) FRCR,
Consultant Radiologist and Clinical Professor of Radiology,
Aberdeen Royal Hospitals NHS Trust, Aberdeen, UK

WB SAUNDERS
An Imprint of Elsevier Science Limited

Reprinted 1998
Reprinted 1999
Reprinted 2000
Reprinted 2001
Reprinted 2002

ISBN 0-7020-1770-1

British Library Cataloguing in Publication Data
A catalogue record for this book is available from the British Library

Library of Congress Cataloging in Publication Data
A catalog record for this book is available from the Library of Congress

Medical knowledge is constantly changing. As new information becomes
available, changes in treatment, procedures, equipment and the use of drugs
become necessary. The authors and Publishers have, as far as it is possible, take
care to ensure that the information given in the text is accurate and up to date.
However, readers are strongly advised to confirm that the information, especiall
with regard to drug usage, complies with latest legislation and standards of
practice.

The Publishers and authors have made every effort to trace the copyright holder
for borrowed material. If they have inadvertently overlooked any, they will be
pleased to rectify the matter at the first opportunity.

Typeset by Phoenix Photosetting, Chatham, Kent
Printed and bound in Great Britain by
Martins the Printers Ltd, Berwick upon Tweed

CONTENTS

PREFACE

While this book has been written primarily for trainee radiologists studying for the FRCR First Examination and the Preface is addressed to them, we expect that the text will be helpful to others interested in medical imaging.

We have avoided complex formulae but some simple equations are used to aid the memory. The ability to sketch graphs, with their axes carefully labelled, can be useful in the examination. Usually it is the shape of the graph that matters, with the scales identified as linear or logarithmic as appropriate. Much of the data in the text is simply illustrative and usually approximate or typical values are given. Imaging technology is advancing continually so the values applicable to equipment and methods in current use in the local radiology department should be known.

Details of the construction of imaging equipment are only given as necessary to understand the nature of the radiation beams and the creation of images. It is important to relate our basic line diagrams to the specific equipment used in the local department. The purpose of various controls and how they affect the image should be known. Practical knowledge and experience are essential. For every imaging procedure, relevant aspects of equipment design, machine settings and the recording media should be observed.

Each method of medical imaging is a compromise between the conflicting requirements of maximizing the information carried by the image (its quality) while minimizing the risk it carries to the patient. This is the theme of the book. Throughout the first five chapters, there are references to factors that affect the patient dose and how it can be minimized. Chapter 6 includes current thinking on radiation hazards and protection, knowledge of which subject is a hallmark of the radiologist.

Various measures of image quality are described including spatial resolution, contrast and quantum noise. These ideas are introduced in Chapters 2 and 3 for 'conventional' radiography with films and screens. They are developed further in Chapters 4 and 5 as the effects are progressively more limiting for fluoroscopic and gamma images. This stepwise approach seemed preferable to a portmanteau chapter devoted to image quality.

A common theme of the later chapters is the production and processing of images by computer. Digital images are first encountered in Chapter 4 and recur in the three chapters on gamma imaging, ultrasound and magnetic resonance imaging (MRI), each of which is relatively self-contained, so that they can be studied in any order. Our descriptions of the various artefacts in digital images, should be related to those seen in real diagnostic images.

Each of the methods of digital imaging depends on two procedures: sampling and fourier transform. These we expand in the final chapter where we also give an approximate treatment of another measure of image quality: modulation transfer function. These are essentially mathematical ideas but can be explained adequately using analogies and graphs.

MRI is a rapidly developing technique. The physics is somewhat complex and the time allocated for its teaching for the First Examination is severely limited. Consequently, we have concentrated on the three basic pulse sequences, the use of gradient fields and safety aspects. Some additional detail is included as background to study for the final examination. MRI is a topic that repays reading several times.

Medical imaging continues to develop through collaboration between radiologists, scientists and engineers from many countries. This can lead to differences in approach and there are often several alternative names and acronyms for the same or similar quantities. We mention most of these to make recognition easier when answering multiple choice and viva questions. At the end of each chapter, there are specimen viva questions, composed by Professor Weir.

Professor Weir also made many valuable suggestions to the manuscript and saved us from a number of radiological solecisms. We are indebted too, to our colleagues in Birmingham and Southampton, particularly, Mr M F Docker, Dr V Gazzard and Dr E A Moore for commenting on various draft chapters. Any imperfections that remain are ours alone. We express our thanks to our publisher, Margaret Macdonald, and the W B Saunders editorial staff; and not least, to generations of students with whose help we have learned so much.

R F Farr
P J Allisy-Roberts

INTRODUCTION

When I was asked to participate in this project, I was initially rather hesitant for two reasons. Firstly, despite being a Part I Fellowship of the Royal College of Radiologists (FRCR) physics examiner in the past, I would regard my knowledge of Medical Physics as 'only reasonable' but certainly insufficient to write a textbook. Secondly, I needed gentle persuasion that this text would add significantly to the literature. However, after becoming involved, I am now delighted to have been convinced, because not only do I know more physics than I thought but, more importantly, I also understand it, as well as having no doubt that this text will make an important contribution to the comprehension of the scientific basis of modern medical imaging.

The authors are both well-known and respected names within medical physics and their combined efforts over the years have led to their desire to impart their knowledge to wider circles than just their own students and lecture programs.

The text is essentially based on the revised medical physics curriculum for Part I of the FRCR examination. There are eight chapters covering all areas with examples of viva questions at the end of each. At the end of the book is extra information on areas that require further understanding, e.g. modulation transfer function, Fourier analysis, etc., that radiologists will find helpful. The revised Part I FRCR syllabus places more strength on the understanding of modern imaging, e.g. ultrasound and magnetic resonance imaging (MRI), while moving away from other subjects, e.g. basic electricity, mathematics, etc. The text has been designed to incorporate these changes. There is also a need, and this is covered in the text, for radiologists to learn applied physics for their final FRCR examination, particularly MRI, where knowledge of specialized sequences and their relationship to pathophysiology are necessary.

Radiation protection, its rules, legislation, and practice are deliberately covered in great detail together with references for further reading. Radiologists and other clinicians are under increasing pressure, quite correctly, to ensure that the use of ionizing radiations is correctly controlled for maximum patient benefit with minimal complications. Adherence to the guidelines outlined in Chapter 6 is therefore important, and any current legislation needs to be understood and acted upon.

I believe the authors have achieved their aims with this textbook and I am pleased at being asked to contribute my clinical radiological knowledge where appropriate.

J Weir

RADIATION PHYSICS

Diagnostic imaging employs radiations – X, gamma, radiofrequency and sound – to which the body is partly but not completely transparent, and it exploits the special properties of a number of elements and compounds. As *ionizing* radiations (X-rays and gamma rays) are used most, it is best to start by discussing the structure of the atom and the production of X-rays.

Table 1.1 Some fundamental particles

	Relative mass	Relative charge	Symbol
Nucleons			
Neutron	1	0	n
Proton	1	+1	p
Extranuclear			
Electron	$\frac{1}{1840}$	−1	e⁻, β^-
Other			
Positron	$\frac{1}{1840}$	+1	e⁺, β^+
Alpha particle	4	+2	α

1.1 STRUCTURE OF THE ATOM

An atom consists mainly of empty space. Its mass is concentrated in a central nucleus which contains a number A of nucleons, where A is called the mass number. The nucleons comprise Z protons, where Z is the atomic number of the element, and so $(A - Z)$ neutrons.

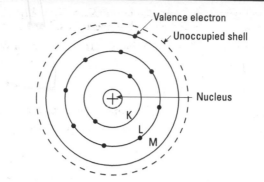

Fig. 1.1 Electron shells in a sodium atom.

A nuclide is a species of nucleus characterized by the two numbers Z and A. The atomic number is synonymous with the name of the element. Thus, $^{12}_{6}C$ refers to a carbon atom with $A = 12$ and $Z = 6$, and is often shortened to ^{12}C and called 'carbon-12'. On the other hand, carbon-14 still has $Z = 6$ but has two more neutrons, which make it unstable and radioactive. It is called a radionuclide.

Orbiting in specific shells around the positively charged nucleus, like planets round the sun, are Z electrons. The shells are designated K, L, M, N, ... outwards from the center. Figure 1.1 illustrates the structure of a sodium atom with two electrons in the K-shell, eight in the L-shell and one in the outermost M-shell.

In each atom, the outermost or *valence* shell is concerned with the chemical, thermal, optical, and electrical properties of the element. X-rays involve the inner shells, and radioactivity concerns the nucleus. Radioactivity is described in Chapter 5, where alpha and beta particles and gamma rays are discussed further.

No valence shell can have more than eight electrons. Metals have one, two, or three valence electrons, one of which is easily detached from the atom and is called 'free'. This accounts for their good conduction of heat and electricity.

Silver bromide is an example of an *ionic crystal*, and consists of equal numbers of positive silver ions (silver atoms which have each lost their single valence electron) and negative bromine ions (bromine atoms which have each gained an outer shell electron). The two kinds of ion hold each other, by electrostatic attraction, in a highly regular three-dimensional lattice. This accounts for the well-known properties of such crystals. Other examples are sodium iodide and cesium iodide.

Binding energy

An atom is said to be *ionized* when one of its electrons has been completely removed. The detached electron is a negative ion and the remnant atom a positive ion. Together they form an ion pair.

The binding energy (E) of an electron in an atom is the energy expended in completely removing the electron from the atom against the attractive force of the positive nucleus. This energy is expressed in electronvolts (eV), explained in Section 1.10.

The binding energy depends on the shell ($E_K > E_L > E_M$ ...), and on the element, increasing as the atomic number increases. For example:

In the case of tungsten (W; $Z = 74$) the binding energies of different shell are

E_K	E_L	E_M
70	11	2 keV

In the case of the K shell, the binding energies of different elements are

W ($Z = 74$)	I ($Z = 53$)	Mo ($Z = 42$)	Cu ($Z = 29$)
70	33	20	9 keV

The binding energy is never greater than 100 keV.

An atom is *excited* when an electron is raised from one shell to another farther out. This involves the expenditure of energy; the atom as a whole has more energy than normal and so is said to be excited. For example, a valence electron can be raised to one of the unoccupied shells farther out, shown dashed in Fig. 1.1. When it falls back, the energy is re-emitted as a single 'packet' of energy or photon of light (visible or ultraviolet). This is an example of the quantum aspects of electromagnetic radiation.

1.2 ELECTROMAGNETIC RADIATION

This is the term given to energy traveling across empty space. All forms of electromagnetic radiation travel with the same velocity (c) as light when *in vacuo*, very close to 3×10^8 m s^{-1} and not significantly less in air. They are named according to the way in which they are produced and the special properties they possess. X-rays (emitted by X-ray tubes) and gamma rays (emitted by radioactive nuclei) have essentially the same properties and differ only in their origin.

Quantum aspects

Electromagnetic radiation can be regarded as a stream of 'packets' or quanta of energy, called photons, traveling in straight lines.

Wave aspects

Electromagnetic radiation can also be regarded as sinusoidally varying electric and magnetic fields, traveling with velocity c when *in vacuo*. They are transverse waves: the electric and magnetic field vectors point at right angles to each other and to the direction of travel of the wave.

At any point, the graph of field strength against *time* is a sine wave, depicted as a solid curve in Fig. 1.2a. The peak field strength is called the amplitude (A). The interval between successive crests of the wave is called the period (T). The frequency (f) is the number of crests passing a point in a second, and $f = 1/T$. The dashed curve refers to a later instant, showing how the wave has travelled forward with velocity c.

At any instant, the graph of field strength against *distance* is also a sine wave (solid curve in Fig. 1.2b). The distance between successive crests of the wave is called the wavelength (λ).

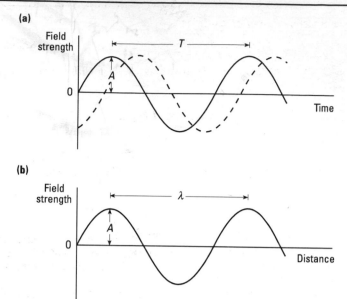

Fig. 1.2 Electromagnetic wave. Field strength versus (a) time and (b) distance.

Table 1.2 Electromagnetic spectrum

	Wavelength	Frequency	Energy
Radio waves	30–6 m	**10–50 MHz**	40–200 neV
Infrared	**10–0.7 μm**	30–430 THz	0.12–1.8 eV
Visible light	**700–400 nm**	430–750 THz	1.8–3 eV
Ultraviolet	**400–100 nm**	750–3000 THz	3–12 eV
X- and gamma	60–2.5 pm	$5 \times 10^6 - 120 \times 10^6$ THz	**20–500 keV**

Typical ranges are in rounded values. The nomenclature that is usually used in practice is emphasized in bold.

Wavelength and frequency are inversely proportional to each other,

$$\text{wavelength} \times \text{frequency} = \text{constant}$$

and is equal to the velocity. This relation is true of all kinds of wave motion, including sound, although for sound the velocity is about a million times less.

The types of radiation are listed in Table 1.2, in order of increasing photon energy, increasing frequency, and decreasing wavelength. When the energy is less than 1 keV the radiation is usually described in terms of its frequency, except that visible light is usually described in terms of its wavelength. It is curious that only radiations at the ends of the spectrum, radio waves and X- or gamma rays, penetrate the human body sufficiently to be used in transmission imaging.

Wave and quantum theories combined

Photon energy is proportional to the frequency. The constant of proportionality is called *Planck's constant (h)*. Thus, $E = hf$.

More usefully, since frequency is inversely proportional to wavelength, so also is photon energy:

$$E \text{ (in keV)} = 1.24/\lambda \text{ (in nm)}$$

For example:

Blue light	$\lambda = 400$ nm	$E \approx 3$ eV
Typical X- and gamma rays	$E = 140$ keV	$\lambda \approx 0.1$ nm

Intensity

Radiation travels in straight lines called rays which radiate in all directions from a point source. A collimated set of rays is called a beam. A beam of radiation can be visualized by taking at some point a cross-section at right angles to the beam (Fig. 1.3a).

Suppose the beam is switched on for a given (exposure) time. Simply counting the photons allows the number per unit area passing through the cross-section in the time to be determined, and is called the *photon fluence* at the point. A beam may contain photons of different energies. Adding up the energies of all the individual photons gives the total amount of energy per unit area passing through the cross-section in the time, and is called the energy fluence at the point.

The total amount of energy per unit area passing through the cross-section *per unit time* (watts per square millimeter) is called the energy fluence rate at the point, and is also referred to as the beam *intensity*. In wave theory, intensity is proportional to the square of the amplitude (A, see Fig. 1.2), measured from the peak of the wave to the axis.

Energy fluence and intensity are not easy to measure directly. As explained in Section 1.8, in the case of X- and gamma rays, an easier indirect measurement of energy fluence is usually made, namely *'air kerma'*; and, instead of intensity, 'air kerma rate'. The relationship between these quantities is discussed in Section 1.10.

Inverse square law

Since electromagnetic radiation travels in straight lines, as Fig. 1.3 shows, the dimensions of the beam are proportional to the distance from a point source S. As a result, the area of the beam is proportional to the square of the distance from a point source. Therefore, in the *absence of scatter and absorption*, the intensity of the radiation is inversely proportional to the square of the distance from a *point source*. Note these conditions which must hold if this, the inverse square law, is to hold.

When the distance is changed:

$$\frac{\text{new intensity}}{\text{old intensity}} = \frac{(\text{old distance})^2}{(\text{new distance})^2}$$

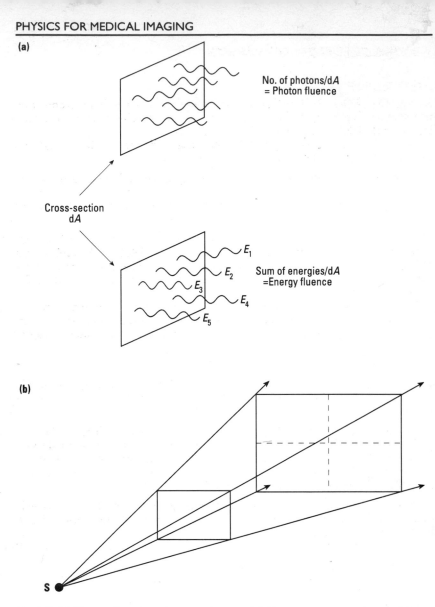

(a)

No. of photons/dA
= Photon fluence

Cross-section
dA

E_1

E_2

E_3

E_4

E_5

Sum of energies/dA
=Energy fluence

(b)

S

Fig. 1.3 (a) Photon fluence and energy fluence. (b) The inverse square law applying to a point source S.

or

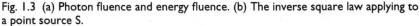

$$\frac{\text{new air kerma rate}}{\text{old air kerma rate}} = \frac{(\text{old distance})^2}{(\text{new distance})^2}$$

Halving the distance quadruples the intensity or air kerma rate; doubling the distance reduces them by a factor of 4, as illustrated in Fig. 1.3b.

1.3 PRODUCTION OF X-RAYS

The X-ray tube

X-rays are produced when fast moving electrons are suddenly stopped by impact on a metal *target*. The kinetic energy of the electrons is converted into X-rays (1%) and into heat (99%).

An X-ray tube, depicted in Fig. 1.4, consists of two electrodes sealed into an evacuated *glass envelope*:

◆ a negative electrode (*cathode*) which incorporates a fine tungsten coil or filament;
◆ a positive electrode (*anode*) which incorporates a smooth flat metal target, usually of tungsten.

The *filament* is heated to incandescence and emits electrons by the process of thermionic emission. At such high temperatures (2200°C) the atomic and electronic motion in a metal is sufficiently violent to enable a fraction of the free electrons to leave the surface, despite the net attractive pull of the lattice of positive ions.

These electrons are then repelled by the negative cathode and attracted by the positive anode. Because of the *vacuum* they are not hindered in any way, and bombard the target with a velocity around half the speed of light.

Kilovoltage and milliamperage

Two sources of electrical energy are required and are derived from the alternating current (AC) mains by means of transformers. Figure 1.4 shows:

◆ The filament heating voltage (about 10 V) and current (about 10 A).
◆ The accelerating voltage (typically 30–150 kV) between the anode and cathode ('high tension', 'kilovoltage', or 'kV'). This drives the current of electrons (typically 0.5–1000 mA) flowing between the anode and cathode ('tube current', 'milliamperage', or 'mA').

The mA is controlled by varying the filament temperature. A small increase in filament temperature, voltage, or current produces a large increase in tube current.

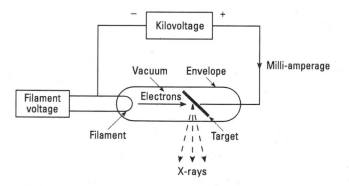

Fig. 1.4 An X-ray tube and its power supplies.

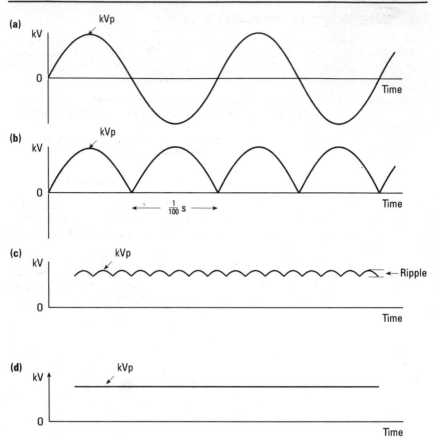

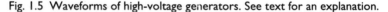

Fig. 1.5 Waveforms of high-voltage generators. See text for an explanation.

An X-ray set is designed so that, unlike most electrical components, increasing or decreasing the tube voltage does not affect the tube current. It is also designed so that the kV is unaffected by changes in the mA. The two factors can therefore be varied independently.

The *waveform* of a high-voltage generator describes a graph showing how voltage varies with time. Figure 1.5 depicts the waveforms of four types of high-tension voltage supply commonly used:

(a) Alternating voltage ('self-rectification').
(b) Pulsating direct current (DC) ('full wave rectified, single-phase').
(c) 'Constant potential', which is steady DC with a small ripple from a 'three-phase' generator; '12 pulse' has a smaller ripple (4%) than '6 pulse' (13%).
(d) High frequency (HF; in which AC of 1 kHz or higher is generated within the set itself), which is steady DC with negligible ripple. HF generators are particularly compact and efficient.

The anode–cathode voltage is often stated as the peak value (kV_p) although in modern generators the terminology 'kV' is more usual.

Processes occurring in the target of an X-ray tube

Each electron arrives at the surface of the target with a kinetic energy (in kiloelectronvolts) equivalent to the kV between the anode and cathode at that instant. The electrons penetrate several micrometers into the target and lose their energy by a combination of processes:

◆ As a large number of very small energy losses, by interaction with the outer electrons of the atoms; constituting unwanted *heat* and causing a rise of temperature.

◆ As large energy losses producing *X-rays*, by interaction with either the inner shells of the atoms or the field of the nucleus.

Interaction with the K-shell: line spectrum, characteristic radiation

As depicted in Fig. 1.6, when an electron (a) from the filament collides with an electron in the K-shell of an atom, an electron (b) will be ejected from the atom, provided that the energy of the bombarding electron is greater than the binding energy of the shell.

The hole so created in the K-shell is most likely to be filled by an electron (c) falling in from the L-shell with the emission of a single X-ray photon (d) of energy equal to the difference in the binding energies of the two shells, $E_K - E_L$. The photon is referred to as K_α radiation.

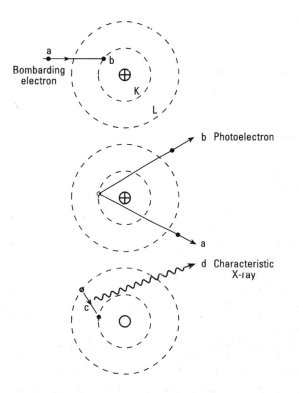

Fig. 1.6 Production of characteristic radiation.

Alternatively, but less likely, the hole may be filled by an electron falling in from the M-shell with the emission of a single X-ray photon of energy $E_K - E_M$, referred to as K_β radiation.

In the case of the usual target material, tungsten ($Z = 74$),

$$E_K = 70 \text{ keV}, E_L = 12 \text{ keV, and } E_M = 2 \text{ keV.}$$

Thus, the K_α radiation has a photon energy of 58 keV and the K_β radiation has a photon energy of 68 keV.

There is also L-radiation, produced when a hole created in the L-shell is filled by an electron falling in from farther out. Even in the case of tungsten these photons have only 10 keV of energy, insufficient to leave the X-ray tube assembly, and so they play no part in radiology.

The X-ray photons produced in an X-ray tube in this way have a few discrete or separate photon energies and constitute a *line spectrum*.

In the case of another target material, molybdenum ($Z = 42$),

$$E_K = 20 \text{ KeV}, E_L = 2.5 \text{ keV}$$

and so the K_α radiation has a photon energy of 17.5 keV and the K_β radiation has a photon energy of nearly 20 keV.

The photon energy of the K-radiation therefore increases as the atomic number of the target increases. It is *characteristic* of the target material and is unaffected by the tube voltage.

A K-electron cannot be ejected and the K-radiation is not produced at all if the peak tube voltage is less than E_K, i.e. 70 kV in the case of a tungsten target. The rate of production of the characteristic radiation increases as the kV is increased above this value.

Interaction with the nucleus: bremsstrahlung, continuous spectrum

As depicted in Fig. 1.7, if a bombarding electron penetrates the K-shell and approaches close to the nucleus it is deflected. It approaches fast and leaves less quickly, losing some or all of its energy. The lost energy is carried away as a single photon of X-rays or bremsstrahlung (literally, 'braking radiation'). Except in mammography, 80% or more of the X-rays emitted by a diagnostic X-ray tube are bremsstrahlung.

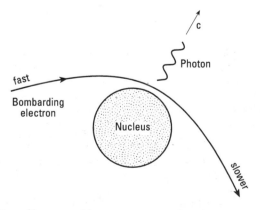

Fig. 1.7 Production of bremsstrahlung.

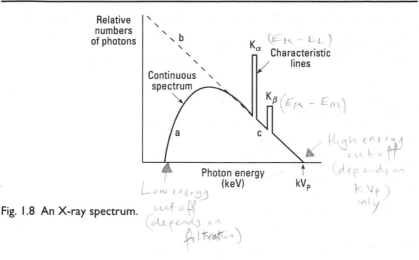

Fig. 1.8 An X-ray spectrum.

Very rarely, an electron arriving at the target is immediately and completely stopped in this way and produces a single photon of energy equivalent to the kV_p. This is the largest photon energy that can be produced at this kilovoltage.

It is more likely that the bombarding electron first loses some of its energy as heat and then, when it interacts with the nucleus, it loses only part of its remaining energy, with the emission of bremsstrahlung of lower photon energy.

The X-rays may be emitted in any direction (although mainly sideways to the electron beam) and with any energy up to the maximum. Figure 1.8 plots the relative number of photons having each photon energy (kiloelectronvolts). The bremsstrahlung forms a *continuous spectrum* (a). The maximum photon energy (kiloelectronvolts) is equivalent to the kV_p.

The dashed line (b) in Fig. 1.8 shows the spectrum of bremsstrahlung produced near the target nuclei, but the target itself, the glass wall of the tube, and other materials collectively referred to as the filtration substantially absorb the lower-energy photons. There is therefore a low-energy cut-off, at about 20 keV, as well as a maximum energy. The latter depends only on the kV_p and the former on the filtration added to the tube (see Section 1.9).

The average or *effective energy* of the continuous spectrum lies between these two, and is typically one-third to one-half of the kV_p. Thus, an X-ray tube operated at 90 kV_p can be thought of as emitting, effectively, 45 keV X-rays. As this peak kV is greater than the K-shell binding energy, characteristic X-rays are also produced. They are shown at c in Fig. 1.8 as lines superimposed on the continuous spectrum.

The area of the spectrum represents the total output of all X-ray photons emitted. Figure 1.9 compares the spectrum from a tube with a tungsten target, operating at three different kV values. As the tube voltage is increased, both the width and height of the spectrum increase. Its area increases and consequently so does the output of X-rays, which is proportional to kV^2.

The *intensity of* X-rays emitted is proportional to $kV^2 \times mA$. (The exact exponent depends on the filtration.) This may be compared with the

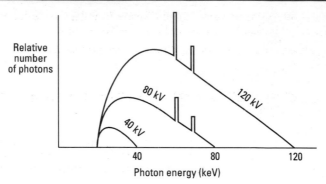

Fig. 1.9 Effect of tube kilovoltage on X-ray spectra.

electrical power supplied, which is proportional to kV × mA. The *efficiency* of X-ray production is the ratio

$$\frac{\text{X-ray output}}{\text{electrical power supplied}}$$

and increases with the kV. The efficiency is greater the higher the atomic number of the target.

Controlling the X-ray spectrum

To summarize, there are five factors affecting the X-ray spectrum. The following are the effects of altering each in turn, the other four remaining constant:

◆ Increasing the kV shifts the spectrum upward and to the right, as shown in Fig. 1.9. It increases the maximum and effective energies and the total number of X-ray photons. Below a certain kV (70 kV for a tungsten target) the characteristic K-radiation is not produced.

◆ Increasing the mA does not affect the shape of the spectrum but increases the output of both bremsstrahlung and characteristic radiation in proportion.

◆ Changing the target to one of lower *atomic number* reduces the output of bremsstrahlung but does not otherwise affect its spectrum, unless the filtration is also changed. The photon energy of the characteristic lines will also be less (Fig. 3.9).

◆ Whatever the kilovoltage *waveform* (see Fig. 1.5) the maximum and minimum photon energies are unchanged. However, a constant potential or three-phase generator produces more X-rays and at higher energies than those produced by a single-phase pulsating potential generator, operating with the same values of kV_p and mA. Both the output and the effective energy of the beam is therefore greater. This is because in Fig. 1.5c,d the tube voltage is at the same peak value throughout the exposure. In Fig. 1.5a,b it is below peak value during the greater part of each half cycle. A single-phase generator produces useful X-rays in pulses, each lasting 30 ms during the middle of each 100 ms half cycle of the mains.

For the effect of the fifth factor, *filtration*, see Section 1.9.

1.4 THE INTERACTION OF X- AND GAMMA RAYS WITH MATTER

Where the following refers to X-rays it applies equally well to gamma rays. Figure 1.10 illustrates the three possible fates of the individual photons when a beam of X- or gamma rays travels through matter. They may be:

- *Transmitted*: pass through unaffected, as primary or direct radiation.
- *Absorbed*: transferring to the matter all of their energy (the photon disappearing completely) or some of it (partial absorption).
- *Scattered*: diverted in a new direction, with or without loss of energy, and so may leave the beam (as scattered or secondary radiation).

X-ray absorption and scattering processes are stochastic processes, governed by the statistical laws of chance. It is impossible to predict which of the individual photons in a beam will be transmitted by 1 mm of a material, but it is possible to be quite precise about the fraction of them that will be, on account of the large numbers of photons the beam contains.

Attenuation

Attenuation refers to the fact that there are fewer photons in the emerging beam than in the beam entering the material:

attenuation = absorption + scatter

In practice, X-ray beams are usually both large and composed of a range (or spectrum) of photon energies. It is helpful to consider first the simpler case.

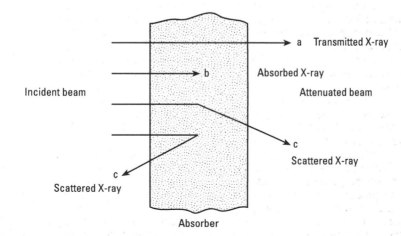

Fig. 1.10 Interaction of X- or gamma rays with matter.

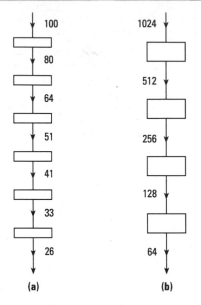

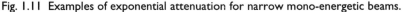

Fig. 1.11 Examples of exponential attenuation for narrow mono-energetic beams.

A narrow, monoenergetic beam of X-rays

The fundamental law of X-ray attenuation states that equal thicknesses of an absorber transmit equal fractions (percentages) of the radiation entering them. This is illustrated in Fig. 1.11a, where each sheet reduces the beam by 20%.

In particular, the *half-value layer* (HVL) is the thickness of stated material which will reduce the intensity of a narrow beam of X-radiation to one-half of its original value.

For example, as in Fig 1.11b, two successive half-value layers reduce the intensity of the beam by a factor $2 \times 2 = 4$. Ten HVLs reduce the intensity of the beam by a factor $2 \times 2 = 4$. Ten HVLs reduce the intensity of the beam by a factor $2^{10} \approx 1000$.

The HVL is a measure of the penetrating power or effective energy of the beam. It is useful to have a parameter which measures the attenuating properties of the material. This is the *linear attenuation coefficient* (μ), which is inversely proportional to the HVL:

$$\mu = 0.69/HVL \quad \text{or} \quad HVL = 0.69/\mu$$

More precisely, the linear attenuation coefficient measures the probability that a photon interacts (i.e. is absorbed or scattered) per unit length of the path it travels in a specified material.

However, the linear attenuation coefficient only applies to narrow monoenergetic beams. The HVL applies only to narrow beams, but they need not be monoenergetic.

The HVL decreases and the linear attenuation coefficient therefore increases as:

◆ the density of the material increases;

14

◆ the atomic number of the material increases;
◆ the photon energy of the radiation decreases.

For example, lead is more effective than either aluminum or tissue at absorbing X-rays because of its higher density and atomic number. X-rays of 140 keV are more penetrating and are said to be 'harder' than those of 20 keV.

The mass attenuation coefficient (μ/ρ) is obtained by dividing the linear coefficient by the density of the material. It is therefore independent of density and depends only on the atomic number and photon energy.

Exponential graph

However thick the absorber, it is never possible to absorb an X-ray beam completely. This is shown, in Fig. 1.12a, by the shape – an exponential curve – of the graph of percentage transmission versus thickness d, both being plotted on linear scales. If, as in Fig. 1.12b the percentage transmission is plotted on a logarithmic scale, a linear graph results, making it easier to read off the HVL and calculate μ.

The experimental arrangement for measuring HVL and the attenuation coefficient is illustrated in Fig. 1.13a. The beam is restricted by means of a lead diaphragm or collimator to just cover a small detector. The diaphragm

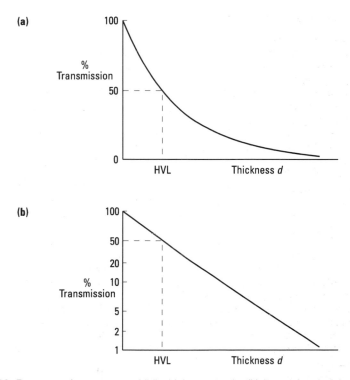

Fig. 1.12 Exponential attenuation; HVL. (a) Linear scale. (b) Logarithmic scale.

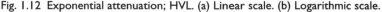

(a)

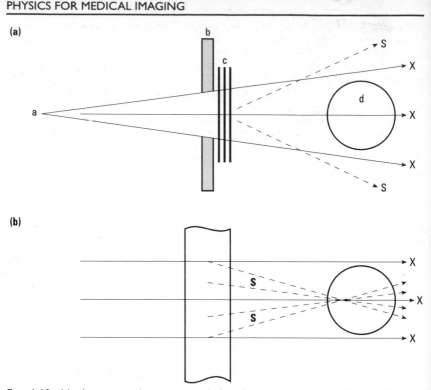

(b)

Fig. 1.13 (a) A narrow beam is used for the measurement of the HVL. (b) Transmission of a wide beam.

b and sheets of the absorbing material c are positioned halfway between the source a and detector d. This arrangement, referred to as 'good geometry', minimizes the amount of scattered radiation SS entering the detector. A second collimator may be placed in front of the detector.

Attenuation of a wide beam

The percentage transmission by the same object of a wide beam of X- or gamma rays is greater than that of a narrow beam of photons of the same energy, for the following reason. In Fig. 1.13a, most of the scatter, such as SS, produced by a narrow beam of radiation XX leaves the beam but, as Fig. 1.13b shows, a wide beam produces more scatter SS and much of it stays within the beam.

Attenuation of a heterogeneous beam

The beams produced by X-ray tubes are heterogeneous (polyenergetic), i.e. they comprise photons of a wide range of energies. As the beam travels through an attenuating material, the lower-energy photons are attenuated proportionally more than the higher-energy photons. The exponential law does not therefore apply exactly. It is still, however, correct to refer to the HVL of the beam. The HVL of a typical diagnostic beam is 30 mm in tissue, 12 mm in bone, and 0.15 mm in lead.

As the beam penetrates the material, it becomes progressively more homogeneous. The proportion of higher-energy photons in the beam increases: a process described as filtration.

The average energy of the photons increases – the beam becomes 'harder' or more penetrating. The 'second HVL', which would reduce the beam intensity from 50 to 25%, is thus greater than the 'first HVL', which reduces it from 100 to 50%.

The X-ray beams used in practice are usually both wide and heterogeneous, and the exponential law of absorption does not strictly apply. However, it is still possible to use the exponential law of X-ray attenuation in approximate calculations together with an effective attenuation coefficient.

Interaction processes

Three processes of interaction between X-rays and matter contribute to attenuation:

◈ interaction with a loosely bound or 'free' electron – the Compton process, also called modified scatter (see Section 1.5);
◈ interaction with an inner shell or 'bound' electron – photoelectric absorption, a disappearance process (see Section 1.6);
◈ interaction with a bound electron – unmodified scatter, also called coherent scatter (see Section 1.10).

1.5 COMPTON PROCESS (MODIFIED SCATTER)

As depicted in Fig. 1.14, the photon bounces off a free electron which recoils, taking away some of the energy of the photon as kinetic energy. The photon is scattered, i.e. diverted in a new direction, with reduced energy.

The angle of scatter θ is the angle between the scattered ray and the incident ray. Photons may be scattered in all directions. The electrons are projected only in sideways and forward directions.

Effect of the angle of scattering

Figure 1.14 illustrates three different angles of scattering. The lengths of the arrows indicate the relative energies of the recoil electrons. It will be seen that the greater the angle of scatter:

◈ the greater the energy and range of the recoil electron, and also
◈ the greater the loss of energy (and increase of wavelength) of the scattered photon.

Thus, a back-scattered photon ($\theta = 180°$) is less energetic or is 'softer' than a side-scattered photon ($\theta = 90°$), which in turn is softer than a forward-scattered photon ($\theta = 0°$).

Effect of initial photon energy

The higher the initial photon energy:

◈ the greater the remaining photon energy of the scattered radiation and the more penetrating it is; also

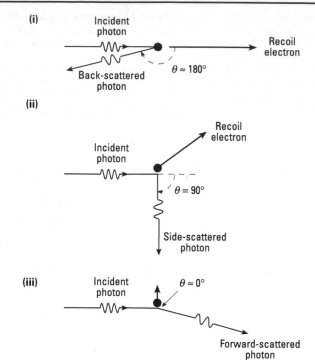

Fig. 1.14 Compton scattering by a free electron.

◆ the greater the energy that is carried off by the recoil electron and the greater its range.

This is seen in the following examples:

Incident photon	Back-scattered photon	Recoil electron
25 keV	22 keV	3 keV
150 keV	100 keV	50 keV

The softening effect of Compton scatter is therefore greatest with large scattering angles as well as with high energy X-rays.

The Compton process contributes to the total linear attenuation coefficient μ, an amount σ which is called the Compton linear attenuation coefficient. The probability σ that the Compton process will occur is proportional to the physical density (mass per unit volume) of the material, as with all attenuation processes. (It is also proportional to electron density, as explained in Section 1.10) It is independent of the atomic number of the material, as it concerns only 'free' electrons. Finally, it decreases only slightly over the range of photon energies encountered in diagnostic radiology, and may be thought of as being very approximately proportional to $1/E$.

To summarize:

σ is proportional to ρ/E and is independent of Z

The mass Compton attenuation coefficient σ/ρ is the same within 10% for such diverse materials as air, tissue, bone, contrast media, and lead. They are all represented by a single curve in Fig. 1.16, which shows how σ/ρ varies with photon energy.

The energy carried off by the recoil electron is said to have been absorbed by the material, and the remainder, carried by the photon, to have been scattered. The Compton process is partial absorption. In the diagnostic range of energies no more than 20% of the energy is absorbed, the rest being scattered.

1.6 PHOTOELECTRIC ABSORPTION

When, as in Fig. 1.15, an X- or gamma ray photon (a) 'collides' with an electron in (say) the K-shell of an atom, it can, if its energy is greater than the binding energy of the shell, eject the electron b from the atom. The photon disappears. Part of its energy, equal to the binding energy of the K-shell, is expended in removing the electron from the atom, and the remainder becomes the kinetic energy (KE) of that electron:

$$\text{KE of the electron} = \text{photon energy} - E_K$$

Less often, the X- or gamma ray photon may interact with an electron in

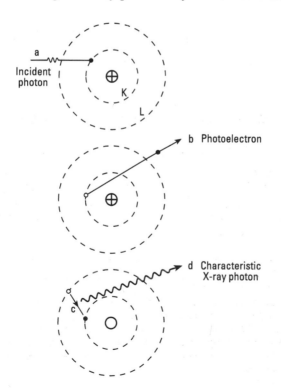

Fig. 1.15 Photoelectric absorption.

the L-shell of an atom. The electron is then ejected from the atom with KE = photon energy − E_L.

The electrons so ejected are called photoelectrons. In each case, the 'holes' created in the atomic shell are filled by electrons falling in from a shell farther out (e.g. electron c in Fig. 1.15), with the emission of a series of photons of characteristic radiation (such as photon d in Fig. 1.15). In this way the whole of the original photon energy is accounted for.

In the case of air, tissue, and other light-atom materials, the characteristic radiation is so soft that it is absorbed immediately with the ejection of a further, low-energy, photoelectron or 'Auger' electron. Thus, all the original photon energy is converted into the energy of electronic motion and is said to have been absorbed by the material. Photoelectric absorption in such materials is complete absorption.

On the other hand, the characteristic rays from barium and iodine in contrast media are sufficiently energetic to leave the patient. In this respect they act like Compton scattered rays.

Photoelectric absorption contributes to the total linear attenuation coefficient μ an amount τ which is called the photoelectric linear attenuation coefficient. Thus $\mu = \sigma + \tau$.

The more tightly the electron is bound to the atom and the nearer the photon energy is to its binding energy, the more likely photoelectric absorption is to happen. And so the probability τ that photoelectric absorption will occur decreases markedly as the photon energy of the radiation increases, being inversely proportional to the cube of the photon energy E. It increases markedly as the atomic number of the material increases, being proportional to the cube of the atomic number Z. Finally, it is proportional to the density of the material, as with all attenuation processes.

To summarize:

$$\tau \propto \rho Z^3/E^3$$

The foregoing is illustrated in Fig. 1.16, which shows how the mass photoelectric attenuation coefficient τ/ρ varies with photon energy in the case of soft tissue (T), having $Z = 7.4$, bone (B), with $Z = 13$, and iodine (I), with $Z = 53$. Note that these graphs are straight lines because logarithmic scales have been used on both axes.

Effective atomic number

A mixture or compound has an effective atomic number which is a (weighted) average of the atomic numbers of the constituent elements. To take account of the photoelectric absorption, the effective atomic number is defined as the cube root of the average of the cube roots of the atomic numbers of the constituents. Some examples are

Fat	Air	Water, muscle	Bone
6	7.6	7.4	13

The Compton and photoelectric interactions depend on the effective atomic number but not on the molecular configuration.

Absorption edges

As the photon energy is increased, photoelectric attenuation decreases according to the above formula until the binding energy E_K of the

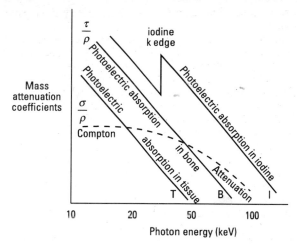

Fig. 1.16 Photoelectric (τ/ρ) and Compton (σ/ρ) mass attenuation coefficients of materials of different atomic numbers at different photon energies.

particular material is reached. At this energy, the photoelectric absorption jumps to a higher value and then decreases again as the photon energy further increases. Called the K-absorption edge, this jump is illustrated for the case of iodine in Fig. 1.16.

This discontinuity is an exception to the general rule that attenuation decreases with increasing energy. The reason is that photons with less energy than E_K can only eject L-electrons and can only be absorbed in that shell. Photons with greater energy than E_K can eject K-electrons as well, and can therefore be absorbed in both shells.

The sudden change of absorption coefficient is called the K-absorption edge, and occurs at different photon energies with different materials. The higher the atomic number of the material, the greater is E_K and the greater is the photon energy at which the edge occurs.

For example, in the case of iodine, $E_K = 33$ keV and photons of energy 31 keV are attenuated much less than photons of energy 35 keV. The K-edges of low atomic number materials such as air, water, tissue, and aluminum have no significance as they occur at $E_K = 1$ keV or less. The absorption edge is important in choosing materials for 'K-edge filters' (see Section 1.9), contrast media (see Section 2.1), and imaging phosphors (see Section 3.1). Since the photon energy of the K-radiation of any material is somewhat less than its E_K, a material is relatively *transparent to its own characteristic radiation.*

Relative importance of Compton and photoelectric attenuation

The photoelectric coefficient is proportional to Z^3/E^3, and is particularly high when the photon energy is just greater than E_K. The Compton coefficient is independent of Z and little affected by E. Accordingly, photoelectric absorption is more important than the Compton process with high-Z materials as well as with relatively low-energy photons. Conversely, the Compton process is more important than photoelectric absorption with low-Z materials as well as with high-energy photons.

For example, there is about a 2% probability that a 30 keV photon traversing 1 mm of soft tissue undergoes a photoelectric interaction. The probability that a photon of this energy undergoes a Compton interaction also happens to be 2%. If a 30 keV photon traverses 1 mm of bone, the probabilities are about 12% and 3%, respectively.

Figure 1.16 compares Compton and photoelectric attenuation for different materials and different photon energies. The photon energy at which the two processes happen to be equally important depends on the atomic number of the material and is about 30 keV for air, water, and tissue, 50 keV for aluminum and bone, 300 keV for iodine and barium, 500 keV for lead.

As regards diagnostic imaging with X-rays (20–140 keV), therefore:

◈ the Compton process is the predominant process for air, water, and soft tissues;
◈ photoelectric absorption predominates for contrast media, lead, and the materials used in films, screens, and other imaging devices; while
◈ both are important for bone.

A third process, which is less important, is mentioned in Section 1.10.

Secondary electrons

The term 'secondary radiation' refers to Compton scattered radiation; and 'secondary electrons' to the recoil electrons and photoelectrons set moving in the material by the two processes. As they travel through the material, the secondary electrons interact with the outer shells of the atoms they pass nearby, and excite or ionize them. The track of the electron is therefore dotted with ion pairs. When traveling through air the electron loses an average of 34 eV per ion pair formed. This is accounted for by about 3 eV being needed to excite an atom and about 10 eV to ionize it, and there being about eight times as many excitations as ionizations.

When it has lost the whole of its initial energy in this way, the electron comes to the end of its *range*. The greater the initial energy of the electron, the greater its range. The range is inversely proportional to the density of the material.

For example, when 140 keV photons are absorbed in soft tissue, some of the secondary electrons are photoelectrons having an energy of 140 keV, able to produce some 4000 ion pairs and having a range of about 0.2 mm.

Most of the secondary electrons are recoil electrons with a spectrum of energies averaging 25 keV and an average range of about 0.02 mm. The ranges in air are some 800 times greater than in tissue. Due to their continual 'collisions' with the atoms, the tracks of secondary electrons are somewhat tortuous.

1.7 PROPERTIES OF X- AND GAMMA RAYS

It is the excitations and ionizations produced by the secondary electrons which account for the various properties of X- and gamma rays:

◈ The ionization of air and other gases makes them electrically conducting: used in the measurement of X- and gamma rays (see Section 1.8).
◈ The ionization of atoms in the constituents of living cells cause biological damage: responsible for the hazards of radiation exposure to

patients and staff and necessitating protection against radiation (see Chapter 6).

◆ The excitation of atoms of certain materials (phosphors) makes them emit light (luminescence, scintillation, or fluorescence): used in the measurement of X- and gamma rays and as a basis of radiological imaging (see Chapters 3, 5 and 6).

◆ The effect on the atoms of silver and bromine in a photographic film leads to blackening (photographic effect): used in the measurement of X- and gamma rays (see Chapter 6) and as a basis of radiography (see Chapter 3).

◆ The greater part of the energy absorbed from an X- or gamma ray beam is converted into increased molecular motion, i.e. heat in the material, and produces an extremely small rise in temperature.

Types of luminescence

When a phosphor absorbs X-rays, the secondary electrons set in motion raise valence electrons to a higher energy level. (The process is similar to that described in Section 1.2 for the excitation of isolated atoms but differs in that each atom in a crystal lattice is affected by the presence of neighboring atoms.) The electrons stay in energy 'traps' and the absorbed energy is stored in the phosphor until the electrons return to the valence shells, with the emission of photons of light.

This may happen spontaneously, either instantaneously in the case of *fluorescence* or after a noticeable interval of time in the case of *phosphorescence*. The latter is called *afterglow* or lag, and is generally to be avoided in imaging.

Or the emission of the light may require stimulation by heat in the case of *thermoluminescence* or by intense light from a laser, in the case of *photostimulation*.

Thermoluminescence is used in measuring radiation dose (see Section 6.9.2), and photostimulation can be used in imaging (computed radiography, see Section 4.4).

Other ionizing radiations

Some ultraviolet radiation has a sufficiently high photon energy to ionize air. Beta particles, emitted by many radioactive substances and other moving electrons (in a television monitor, for example) also possess the above properties. Alpha rays (helium nuclei ^{4}He), (which are particularly stable combinations of two neutrons and two protons) are also emitted by some radioactive substances. Both alpha and beta rays are charged particles and are *directly ionizing*.

X- and gamma rays are *indirectly ionizing*, through their secondary electrons; the 'secondary' ions produced along the track of a secondary electron being many times more than the single 'primary' ionization caused by the initial Compton or photoelectric interaction. Neutrons also ionize tissue indirectly through the hydrogen nuclei they collide with.

I.8 ABSORBED DOSE

The effects of ionizing radiations described above may be correlated with the energy deposited as ionization and excitation of the atoms of the material irradiated. The absorbed dose is the energy deposited per unit mass of the stated material (in joules per kilogram). The SI unit of absorbed dose is the gray (Gy); 1 Gy $= 1$ J kg^{-1}. Dose rate is measured in grays per second, with the usual multiples and submultiples. The concept of absorbed dose applies to all kinds of directly and indirectly ionizing radiations and to any material. It is particularly valuable when considering tissue and biological effects. Whenever the term 'dose' is used in this text, it is taken to mean absorbed dose in the material specified.

Before 1980 the international unit of absorbed dose was the rad. It is still used in many American textbooks, and the conversion factor is 1 Gy $= 100$ rad; 1 rad $= 1$ cGy $= 10$ mGy.

Kerma

Another quantity sometimes used is kerma, which is also measured in grays and can be taken as more or less synonymous with absorbed dose. Kerma is the kinetic energy (of the secondary electrons) *released* per unit mass of irradiated material. Whereas absorbed dose is the energy *deposited* (as ionization and excitation) by the same secondary electrons. In most radiodiagnostic situations they are equal and, in the subject matter of this text, dose and kerma can be used interchangeably.

Measurement of X- and gamma ray dose

It is extremely difficult to measure dose in solids or liquids directly, and it is usual first to measure the dose delivered to air (or 'air kerma') under the same conditions and to multiply it by a conversion factor to obtain the dose in the material. The conversion factor:

$$\frac{\text{dose in stated material}}{\text{dose in air}}$$

depends on the relative amounts of energy absorbed in air and the material.

Like the mass absorption coefficients, the factor depends on the effective atomic number of the material and on the effective energy of the X- or gamma rays. For X-rays used in radiology, the following are approximate values of the factor:

- for muscle, the atomic number of which is not very different to that of air and in which the Compton process predominates, the ratio is close to unity and only varies between 1.0 and 1.1 over the kilovoltage range;
- for compact bone, with its higher atomic number and in which photoelectric absorption is important, the ratio varies from about 4.5 at low kiloelectronvolt energies to 1.2 at high kiloelectronvolt energies;
- for fat, with its lower atomic number the ratio varies in the opposite direction, from about 0.6 at low kiloelectronvolt energies to 1.1 at high kiloelectronvolt energies;
- for the soft tissue elements in cavities within bone (osteocytes, Haversian system, and bone marrow) the ratio lies between those for bone and muscle, and depends on the size of the cavity as well as on the photon energy.

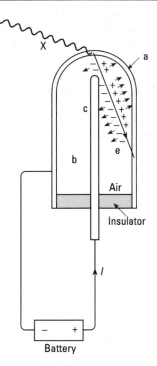

Fig. 1.17 Thimble or cavity ionization chamber.

Thimble or cavity chamber

The *air dose* or kerma can be measured by placing at the point in question a plastic 'thimble' (a), depicted in Fig. 1.17, containing a small mass of air (b), which is indirectly ionized by the X-radiation. Each X-ray photon (X) absorbed in the wall liberates a secondary electron (e), which produces ion pairs along its track. (Although in the diagram the track is for simplicity idealized as a straight line, it is, in fact, quite tortuous.) For each ion pair, 34 eV of energy will have been deposited. Therefore, for each coulomb of charge (either positive or negative) carried by all the ions produced, 34 J of energy will have been deposited.

To measure the charge, the ions are separated before they can recombine by applying a polarizing voltage between the outer thimble wall and a thin central electrode (c). The positive ions are attracted to the negative electrode, and the negative ions (electrons) to the positive electrode. An ionization current I flows, proportional to the dose rate of the radiation and the mass of air in the chamber. The charge can be collected, and the air kerma indicated on a meter or digital read-out. Alternatively, the current can be measured and the air kerma rate similarly indicated.

A polarizing voltage of 100 V is usually sufficient to collect all the ions and produce a 'saturation current'. If the voltage is too low, some of the positive and negative ions recombine, and the ionization current measured is too low. Above a certain 'saturation' voltage, all the ions are separated, and the ionization current is constant, independent of the polarizing (collecting) voltage.

Air has been chosen as the standard material for dosimetry because:

◆ it has an effective atomic number (7.6) close to that of tissue (7.4), so that the conversion factor is close to unity and the conversion of dose in air to dose in tissue can be made easily and accurately;

◆ it is applicable to the measurement of a wide range of X- and gamma ray photon energies;

◆ large and small doses and large and small dose rates are easily and accurately measured;

◆ air is readily available, cheap, universal, and has an invariable composition.

Wall material

The chamber wall must be made of a suitable material.

As Fig. 1.17 shows, the air in the thimble is ionized by secondary electrons which have been set moving by X-rays absorbed in the wall and electrode. So far as the X-rays and their secondary electrons are concerned, these components must be indistinguishable from air, except in density. They must be made of *air-equivalent material*.

An air-equivalent material matches air as regards effective atomic number, and so absorbs energy from an X-ray beam, whatever its energy, to the same extent as the same mass of air. The density is not important; it can conveniently be a solid. There are other conditions to be fulfilled, and a specially compounded plastic may be used.

A simpler alternative is to make the thimble wall (a) of plastic ($Z = 6$), made conducting by an internal coat of graphite, and the inner electrode (c) of a suitably thin aluminum wire ($Z = 13$). By adjusting the length of the wire, the average or effective atomic number of the combination can be made equal to that of air. The chamber is said to be 'air wall' or, since it truly measures the air dose whatever the photon energy of the radiation, apparently *'energy-independent'*. However, corrections are needed, as discussed below.

Wall thickness

The chamber wall must be sufficiently thick.

The dosemeter is designed to measure the air dose at, effectively, a point, namely the center of the thimble. The overall dimensions should therefore be small. Typical values are length 17 mm, diameter 7 mm, and wall thickness 0.7 mm. The larger the air volume, the more sensitive the dosemeter. A 30 ml chamber is often used to check the output of an X-ray set and an even larger one to measure the low-intensity stray radiation near an X-ray set or in a radionuclide calibrator to assess radioactivity (see Section 5.6).

If the wall is too thin, electrons which have been set moving by the X-rays at points in the surroundings can penetrate into the air cavity and contribute to the ionization, giving a false reading.

The wall thickness should be greater than the maximum range of the secondary electrons set in motion by the hardest X-rays to be measured (0.2 mm for the photoelectrons from 140 keV X-rays, for example). Then the ionization is unaffected by the X- and gamma dose rate at points outside the thimble. However, if the wall is too thick it attenuates unduly the radiation being measured.

Energy dependence: correction factors

In practice, the dosemeter is likely to give an incorrect measure of the air dose for two reasons: (1) it is not possible to make the wall and electrode exactly air-equivalent; (2) The X- or gamma rays being measured are attenuated by the walls of the chamber, thus reducing the reading, particularly when measuring low-energy X-rays. Accordingly, the dosemeter reading has to be multiplied by a correction factor, N, which varies with the photon energy, i.e. the dosemeter is 'energy-dependent'.

Another correction has to be applied if the ambient temperature or pressure differ from standard values. If the pressure is too high or if the temperature is too low, air will leak out of the chamber, and the reading will be too low; and vice versa. Such a correction is not needed with sealed chambers.

Standard, free air chamber

The correction factor N is measured at a national standards laboratory (such as the National Physical Laboratory in the UK), where the thimble dosemeter is compared with a standard instrument, the free air chamber. This is designed to measure air dose exactly, whatever the energy of the radiation. The 'wall' of the chamber is ordinary air, and so its 'thickness' has to be some 800 times that appropriate for a thimble chamber. This makes it a very large chamber which is inconvenient for departmental use.

Sealed parallel plate chambers

These are mounted on the light beam diaphragm for measuring the product (air kerma × area of beam). This is easier to measure than the skin dose and is also a better index of the risk to the patient. It effectively measures the total energy entering the patient, most of which is deposited in the tissues, although some re-emerges as scatter. It is referred to as a kerma-area or dose-area product monitor. This chamber must be transparent to light and to X-rays. It must be broader than the widest beam of X-rays used. It must not cast a shadow on the film, and is made of Perspex. The electrodes are made conducting by a transparent layer, a few atoms thick, of a metal such as gold.

Another type of sealed parallel plate chamber can be inserted between the patient and the film cassette for automatic exposure control (see Section 3.8).

Exposure

Not all dosemeters in current use are calibrated to read air kerma in grays. Some are calibrated to read exposure, which is defined as

$$\frac{\text{ionization charge collected}}{\text{mass of air in the thimble chamber}}$$

The obsolescent quantity 'exposure' only applies to X- and gamma rays and not to alpha particles, beta particles, or neutrons, whereas air kerma applies to them all. The SI unit of exposure is coulombs per kilogram:

$$\text{absorbed dose to air (Gy)} = 34 \times \text{exposure (C kg}^{-1})$$

The factor 34 is numerically equal to the energy in electronvolts expended per ion pair.) An older unit of exposure is the roentgen (R). In reading the earlier literature, 'roentgen' can be taken as roughly synonymous with 'rad' or 10 mGy.

Other dosemeters

It is often convenient to measure radiation dose by means of:

- the photographic effect in silver bromide, used in a film badge (see Section 6.9.1);
- the fluorescent effect in sodium iodide, used in a scintillation counter (see also the gamma camera, Section 5.3);
- the thermoluminescence in lithium fluoride, used in a 'TLD' (see Section 6.9.2);
- the photoconductivity in germanium or silicon, used in an 'electronic' dosemeter.

The first two employ materials having a high atomic number, are highly energy dependent, and need calibration against an air wall thimble chamber. Lithium fluoride is sufficiently air or tissue equivalent to be adequate for the measurement of patient and staff doses.

An *electronic dosemeter* consists of a small semiconducting crystal in series with a battery and a digital measuring device. X-rays absorbed by the crystal make it conduct an electric current which is proportional to the dose rate.

Phantoms

When measuring the dose delivered to a patient, the latter is often substituted by a phantom of the same general size and shape as the relevant part of the body and made of tissue-equivalent material. This is a material which matches tissue as regards density and effective atomic number. It therefore absorbs and scatters an X-ray beam, whatever its energy, in the same manner and to the same extent as the same volume of tissue. These conditions are most easily met by water in a thin-walled plastic container. Alternatively, specially compounded rubber or waxes may be used. Phantoms used in mammography are often based on Perspex, which attenuates the X-ray beam more than the same thickness of tissue, for which allowance must be made.

1.9 FILTRATION

When a radiograph is taken, the lower-energy photons in the X-ray beam are mainly absorbed by and deposit dose in the patient. Only a small fraction, if any, reach the film and contribute to the image. The object of filtration is to remove a large proportion of the lower-energy photons before they reach the skin. This reduces the dose received by the patient while hardly affecting the radiation reaching the film, and so the resulting image.

This dose reduction is achieved by interposing between the X-ray tube and patient a uniform flat sheet of metal, usually aluminum, and called the *added* or *additional filtration*. The predominant attenuation process should be photoelectric absorption, which varies inversely as the cube of the photon energy. The filter will therefore attenuate the lower-energy photons (which mainly contribute to patient dose) much more than it does the higher-energy photons (which are mainly responsible for the image).

The X-ray photons produced in the target are first filtered by the window of the tube housing, the insulating oil, the glass insert, and, principally, the target material itself. The combined effect of these disparate components are expressed as an equivalent thickness of aluminum, typically 0.5–1 mm Al and called the *inherent filtration*. The light beam diaphragm mirror also adds to the filtration. When inherent filtration must be minimized, a tube with a window of beryllium ($Z = 4$) instead of glass may be used.

The *total filtration* is the sum of the added filtration and the inherent filtration. For general diagnostic radiology it should be at least 2.5 mm Al equivalent. (This will produce an HVL of about 2.5 mm Al at 70 kV, and 4.0 mm at 120 kV.) Mammography (see Section 3.10) is a special case.

Choice of filter material

The atomic number should be sufficiently high to make the energy-dependent attenuating process, photoelectric absorption, predominate. It should not be too high, since the whole of the useful X-ray spectrum should lie on the high-energy side of the absorption edge. If not, the filter might actually soften the beam.

Aluminum ($Z = 13$) is generally used, as it has a sufficiently high atomic number to be suitable for most diagnostic X-ray beams. With the higher kV values, copper ($Z = 29$) is sometimes used, being a more efficient filter, but it emits 9 kcV characteristic X-rays. These must be absorbed by a 'backing filter' of aluminum on the patient side of the 'compound filter'. Other filter materials (molybdenum or palladium) have absorption edges (20 or 24 keV, respectively) favorable for mammography (see Section 3.10). Erbium (58 keV) has been used at moderate kV values, and is another so-called '*K-edge filter*'.

Effects of filtration

Figure 1.18 shows the spectrum of X-rays generated at 60 kV after passing through 1, 2, and 3 mm aluminum. A filter attenuates the lower-energy X-rays more in proportion than the higher-energy X-rays. It therefore increases the penetrating power (HVL) of the beam at the cost of reducing

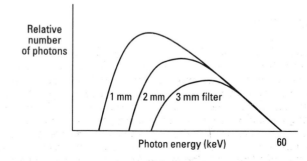

Relative number of photons

1 mm 2 mm 3 mm filter

Photon energy (keV)   60

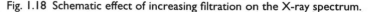

Fig. 1.18 Schematic effect of increasing filtration on the X-ray spectrum.

its intensity. It reduces the skin dose to the patient while having little effect on the radiological image. It is responsible for the low-energy cut-off of the X-ray spectrum, depicted in Figs 1.8 and 1.18.

Increasing the filtration has the following effects. It causes the continuous X-ray spectrum to shrink and move to the right, as seen in Fig. 1.18. It increases the minimum and effective photon energies but does not affect the maximum photon energy. It reduces the area of the spectrum and the total output of X-rays. Finally, it increases the exit dose/entry dose ratio, or film dose/skin dose ratio.

Above a certain thickness, there is no gain from increasing the filtration, as the output is further reduced with little further improvement in patient dose or HVL.

Compensating or wedge filter

A shaped filter may be attached to the tube to make the exposure across the film more uniform and compensate for the large difference in transmission by, for example, the upper and lower thorax, neck and shoulder, or foot and ankle. Similarly, a compensating filter may sometimes be used in mammography (see Section 3.10).

Quantity and quality

The intensity or air kerma rate of an X-ray beam is:

- proportional to the square of the kV;
- greater for a constant potential than a pulsating potential;
- proportional to the mA;
- decreases as the filtration is increased;
- inversely proportional to the square of the distance F from the target;
- greater for high rather than low atomic number targets.

The energy fluence or air kerma is, in addition,

- proportional to the exposure time:

$$\text{dose rate} \propto kV^2 \times mA/F^2 \qquad \text{dose} \propto kV^2 \times mAs/F^2$$

where mAs is milliampere-seconds (i.e. the charge).

The *quality* or penetrating power of an X-ray beam may be specified as the HVL of the beam in a stated material, usually aluminum with diagnostic X-rays.

Alternatively, the quality may be described by the average or *effective energy* of the X-ray spectrum. This may be deduced from the measured HVL. The greater the HVL the greater the effective energy. The effective energy can be defined as the photon energy of monoenergetic X-rays which have the same HVL as the polyenergetic beam being assessed. For example, 100 kV X-rays filtered with 2 mm Al have the same HVL (3 mm Al) as 30 keV photons. When filtered with 10 mm Al the effective energy is increased to 50 keV.

The HVL and effective energy of an X-ray beam:

- increase as the applied kV is increased;
- are greater for constant potential than pulsating potential;
- are unaffected by the mA or exposure time;
- increase as the filtration is increased;
- are unaffected by the distance from the target.

A 'hard' X-ray beam is produced by a high kV and a thick filter; a 'soft' beam by a low kV and a thin filter. Since the two principal factors affecting HVL or effective energy are kV and filtration, and since the latter is normally not changed, it is common in radiography to describe the quality of X-rays simply by stating the tube kV.

1.10 APPENDIX

Units

The SI units of energy and power are the joule (J) and the watt (W): 1 W = 1 J s⁻¹.

The SI units of electric charge and current are the coulomb (C) and ampere (A): 1 A = 1 C s⁻¹ and 1 C = 1 As. A smaller unit of current is the milliampere (mA). A smaller unit of charge is the milliampere-second (mAs).

The SI unit of electrical potential difference (PD) and electromotive force (EMF) is the volt (V). When a charge of 1 C passes through an EMF of 1 V it acquires 1 J of energy.

A smaller unit of energy is the electronvolt (eV), which is the energy acquired by a single electron when it passes through an EMF of 1 V. There are as many electronvolts in a joule as there are electrons in a coulomb (≈ 6.25×10^{18}).

Multiplying factors

Pico-	Nano-	Micro-	Milli-	Kilo-	Mega-	Giga-	Tera-
(p)	(n)	(μ)	(m)	(k)	(M)	(G)	(T)
10^{-12}	10^{-9}	10^{-6}	10^{-3}	10^{3}	10^{6}	10^{9}	10^{12}

Phase

Much use of this important idea will be made in Chapters 7 and 8. It can be illustrated by some simple examples.

The tyre valves of a pair of auto wheels rotate at the same speed but they usually reach their highest point at different times. They are out of step or 'out of phase'. They maintain a constant 'phase difference', which is their angular separation and lies between 0 and 360°. Two objects are said to move in synchronism when their phase difference is constant or, more usually, zero.

The two sine waves in Fig. 1.2a are similarly out of phase. They have the same period or frequency but the dashed curve lags behind the solid curve, reaching its maximum at a later time. They maintain a constant phase difference, which is the time interval between their peaks. It is, however, usually expressed as an angle, lying between 0 and 360°, on a scale which makes the period T correspond to 360°.

In an ordinary single-phase mains supply, the current, carried along a single pair of wires, rises and falls as a single sine wave. In a three-phase supply (referred to in Sections 1.3 and 2.7) the current, carried along three sets of wires, rises and falls as three sine waves having phase differences of 120°.

Electron density

In point of fact, the probability of the Compton process depends on the number of electrons per unit *volume* while being otherwise independent of atomic number. It therefore depends upon

mass per unit volume × No. of electrons per unit mass

The former is the usual 'physical' density and the latter is called the 'electron density'.

Since the number of atoms per unit mass is $\propto 1/A$, and the number of electrons per atom is $\propto Z$, the number of electrons per unit mass must be $\propto Z/A$.

Apart from hydrogen (for which $Z/A = 1$), almost all light elements relevant to radiology have $Z/A = 0.5$. As a result, hydrogenous materials have slightly more electrons per gram than materials without a hydrogen content. The electron density of bone, air, fat, muscle, and water does not vary by more than 10%. On account of this small variation we often simply say that Compton attenuation is proportional to physical density.

Air-equivalent materials and tissue-equivalent materials must have the same electron density as air and soft tissue, respectively; as well as having the properties stated in Section 1.8.

Unmodified scatter

There is a third process whereby X- and gamma rays interact with matter.

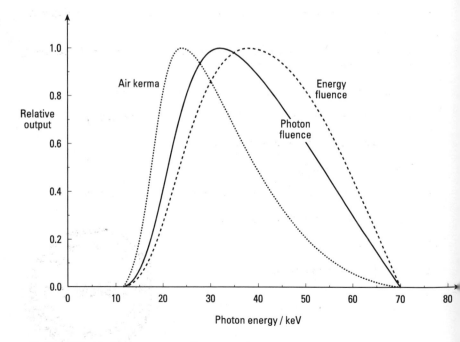

Fig 1.19 Photon fluence, energy fluence, and air kerma distributions.

The photon bounces off an electron which is firmly bound to its parent atom. The atom is too massive to recoil and the photon is scattered with no loss of energy. No secondary electron is set moving and no ionization or other effect is produced in the material. This process occurs only with low-energy photons and at very small angles of scattering, in which case the scattered radiation does not leave the beam and so unmodified scatter has little significance for the radiologist. (It is also known variously as coherent, classical, elastic, or Thomson scattering.)

Photon and energy fluence and air kerma

The relative (spectral) distributions of these three quantities are shown in Fig. 1.19 for a typical 70 kV X-ray beam. By way of example, consider a beam of photons of energy 30 keV. An air kerma of 20 mGy at a point is produced by an energy fluence of about 1 μJ mm^{-2}, which corresponds to a photon fluence of 300 million photons mm^{-2}.

VIVA QUESTIONS

1. What are the photoelectric and Compton effects?

2. What are absorption edges?

3. What relevance does the atomic number 'Z' of an element have to diagnostic imaging?

4. Explain the meaning of (a) the output of an X-ray tube, (b) the half-value layer, and (c) the attenuation coefficient.

5. Compare and contrast a molybdenum target with a tungsten target.

6. What is filtration, how does it work, and what materials are used?

7. How is characteristic radiation produced?

8. What is bremsstrahlung?

9. What are the differences between half wave and full wave rectification?

10. What is the unit of absorbed dose?

11. What is 'kerma'?

12. Explain the inverse square law.

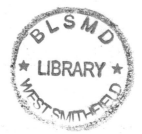

2

IMAGING WITH X-RAYS

2.1 ATTENUATION OF X-RAYS BY THE PATIENT

In conventional projection radiography, a fairly uniform, featureless beam of X-radiation falls on the patient and is differentially absorbed by the tissues of the body. Emerging from the patient, the X-ray beam carries a pattern of intensity which is dependent on the thickness and composition of the organs in the body. Superimposed on the absorption pattern is an overall pattern of scattered radiation.

The X-rays emerging from the patient are captured on a large flat phosphor screen. This converts the invisible X-ray image into a visible image of light, which then is either:

- recorded as a negative image on film, to be viewed on a light box (illuminator); or
- displayed as a positive image on a video monitor.

In this chapter, we consider the invisible X-ray image and some consequences of the properties of X-rays described in the previous chapter, namely:

- they travel in straight lines; and
- they are absorbed and scattered when traveling through matter.

Limiting patient dose

The film–screen or any other imaging system used to convert the X-rays into light requires a specific or minimum dose to produce a satisfactory image. (About 1 µGy per radiograph when using sensitive rare earth screens; 1 µGy or less per second of fluoroscopy.)

This is the exit dose emerging from the patient. The entrance dose, that to the skin proximal to the tube, has to be much higher because of the high attenuation of X-rays by the patient. It might be roughly 10 times greater for a posteroanterior chest, 100 for an anteroposterior abdomen or skull, and 1000 for a lateral pelvis. The average dose lies somewhere between the entrance and exit doses. (The *effective dose*, for reasons given in Chapter 6, is smaller.)

One of the limiting factors in X-ray imaging is the acceptable dose of radiation that can be delivered to the patient. Patient dose should be as small as possible, consistent with producing an image satisfactory for clinical purposes.

Effect of tube kilovoltage on patient dose

Using a higher kilovoltage (kV) makes the beam more penetrating and increases the proportion of high-energy photons which reach the film–screen. As a result, a lower entrance dose is needed for the same exit dose. Increasing the kV therefore reduces the skin dose incurred in producing a satisfactory image and, to a lesser extent, the dose to deeper tissues.

Whereas (see Section 1.3) the output of the X-ray tube and the skin dose rate are roughly proportional to kV^2, the film–screen dose is more nearly proportional to kV^4. (The exponent is 3–5, dependent on patient thickness and field size.)

Effect of focus–film distance on patient dose

Increasing the focus–film distance (FFD) reduces the dose to the patient. This is illustrated in Fig. 2.1. In delivering a specific dose to the film–screen AB, a sufficient number of photons need to enter the skin. At the shorter FFD, with the focal spot at T′, they are concentrated onto a smaller surface area C′D′ and produce a higher skin dose; while at the

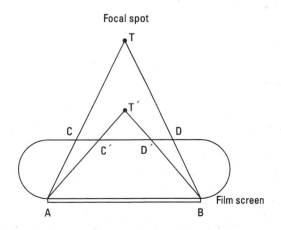

Fig. 2.1 Effect of focus–film distance on patient dose.

longer FFD, with the focal spot at T, they are spread over a larger surface area CD and produce a lower skin dose.

Thus, while increasing the FFD necessitates increasing the charge (milliampere-seconds, mAs) in order to produce the desired number of photons at the film–screen, it nevertheless reduces the skin dose incurred in producing an acceptable image, and to a lesser extent the dose to deeper tissues.

Increasing *filtration* also reduces the skin dose in spite of the fact that an increase in mAs is needed. These ideas are emphasized in Section 6.8 and Table 6.4. Skin dose of course increases linearly with mAs.

Subject contrast

A structure in the patient is demonstrated by two things:

◈ the *resolution, sharpness*, or lack of blurring of the image of its boundary (see Section 2.5); and
◈ the *contrast* between it and adjacent tissues caused by differences in the transmission of X-rays.

We study contrast first, with the aid of a very simple example. Figure 2.2a shows a single structure 1 (say, bone, contrast medium, or gas) surrounded by another material 2 (say, soft tissue). Figure 2.2b shows the pattern of X-rays 'seen' in the image. Contrast in the pattern of X-rays leaving the subject compares E_1, the intensity or dose rate of the rays which have passed through such a structure and E_2, the intensity of those which have passed through the adjacent tissue. All the rays suffer the same attenuation by the tissue layers lying above and below the structure. Contrast is due to the differential attenuation by the structure of thickness t and by an equal thickness of the adjacent tissues.

Accordingly, subject contrast C depends on:

◈ the thickness t of the structure and
◈ the difference in linear attenuation coefficients, μ_1 and μ_2, of the tissues involved.

Thus

$$C \propto (\mu_1 - \mu_2)t$$

So the thicker the structure the greater the contrast. As attenuation depends on tissue density and atomic number, the more the two tissues differ in these respects the greater the contrast. The higher the kV, the smaller the attenuation coefficients and the less the contrast.

Figure 2.3 shows how the linear attenuation coefficient depends on photon energy in the case of air, fat, muscle, bone, and iodine contrast medium. It will be seen that:

◈ the contrast C between bone ($Z = 13$) and muscle, which is proportional to the vertical distance between the two curves, is large and decreases noticeably when the tube kV is increased, due to the effect of photelectric absorption in bone;
◈ the same is true of the contrast between iodine contrast media and soft tissue;
◈ the contrast between the low atomic number tissues, fat ($Z = 6$) and muscle ($Z = 7.4$), is small and does not decrease very much when the tube kV is increased;
◈ the contrast between air and tissue, which have similar atomic numbers, is due to the large difference in density.

(a)

Primary radiation

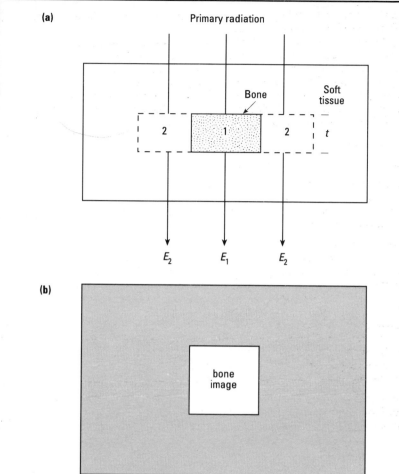

(b)

Fig. 2.2 Primary contrast. (a) X-radiation passing through a single structure I (e.g. bone) that is surrounded by another material 2 (e.g. soft tissue). (b) The X-ray image obtained.

Contrast media

One of the problems in radiography is the low contrast between soft tissues. One way of increasing contrast is to use a lower kV; another is to use a contrast medium. Radioopaque media are chosen to have a sufficiently high atomic number to maximize photoelectric absorption. Ideally, the absorption edge should lie just to the left of the major part of the spectrum of X-rays leaving the patient. Figure 2.3 shows that this is the case with iodine ($Z = 53$, $E_K = 33$ keV). Barium ($Z = 56$, $E_K = 37$ keV) also has a favorably placed absorption edge, and in addition a high density. Contrast media are compounds of one or other of these elements. Air and other gases, the use of which as contrast

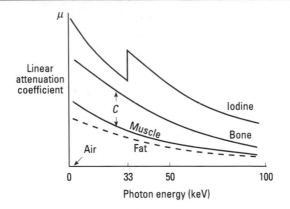

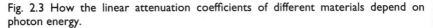

Fig. 2.3 How the linear attenuation coefficients of different materials depend on photon energy.

media has been superseded by computed tomography and magnetic resonance imaging, relied on their low density.

2.2 EFFECT OF SCATTERED RADIATION

The primary radiation carries the information to be imaged, while the scattered radiation obscures it. This is similar to the way in which the light in a room affects the image seen on a television screen. The amount (S) of scattered radiation reaching a point on the film–screen may be several times the amount (P) of primary radiation reaching the point. The ratio S/P depends on the thickness of the part and the area of the beam. The ratio is typically 4:1 for a posteroanterior chest (in which case only 20% of the photons recorded by the film–screen carry useful information) and 9:1 for a lateral pelvis.

Since the scattered radiation is more or less uniform over the image, it acts like a veil and reduces the contrast which would otherwise be produced by the primary rays by the factor $(1 + S/P)$, which may be anything up to 10 times.

This is illustrated in Fig. 2.4a, which shows the same structure as in Fig. 2.2a, while Fig. 2.4b shows the pattern of X-rays 'seen' in the image. If, however, the structure is very close to the film, as in Fig. 2.4c, the scattered rays help to form the image and the contrast is not so greatly reduced.

2.2.1 Scatter reduction and contrast improvement

Measures to reduce the amount of scatter produced by the patient (relative to primary)

◆ *Field size.* Reducing the field area, by the use of cones or the light beam diaphragm, reduces the volume of scattering tissue and so decreases scatter and improves contrast.

◆ *Compression of the patient.* This moves overlying tissues laterally, and reduces the volume of scattering tissue and so decreases scatter and improves contrast.

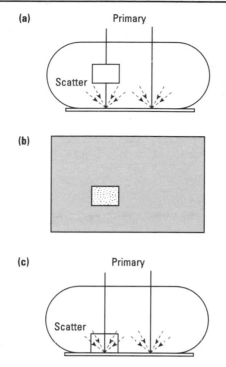

Fig. 2.4 Effects of scattered rays on contrast. (a) The same structure as in Fig. 2.2a. (b) The X-ray pattern seen in the image, with reduced contrast owing to scatter. (c) Moving the structure very close the the film improves contrast as the scattered rays now help to form the imaging.

These first two measures happily also reduce the effective dose to the patient but, use of the following four methods of scatter control require an increase in mAs thus carrying a penalty of increased patient dose and tube loading.

◆ *Kilovoltage*. Using a lower kV produces less forward scatter and more side scatter. At the same time it produces less penetrating scatter, so scatter produced at some distance from the film is less likely to reach it. In practice, these effects may not be very significant. Reducing the kV does increase the contrast, but primarily because of the increased differential photoelectric absorption.

Measures to reduce the amount of scatter after it has left the patient

The amount of scatter (relative to the primary rays) reaching the film–screen may be reduced and contrast increased by interposing between it and the patient:

◆ *A grid*. An 'antiscatter' grid, seen in cross-section in Fig. 2.5, consists of thin (0.07 mm) strips of a heavy metal (such as lead) sandwiched between thicker (0.18 mm) strips of interspace material (plastic, carbon

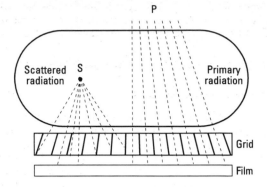

Fig 2.5 Focused grid.

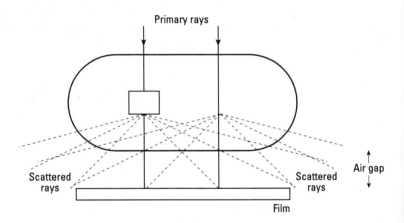

Fig. 2.6 Use of an air gap between the patient and the film–screen.

fiber, or aluminum, which are transparent to X-rays), encased in aluminum or carbon fiber. As described in Section 2.3, the grid acts like a Venetian blind. The lead strips absorb (say, 90% of) the scattered rays which hit the grid obliquely, while allowing (say, 70% of) the primary rays to pass through the gaps and reach the film.

    An air gap. If, as in Fig. 2.6, the film–screen is moved some 30 cm away from the patient, much of the obliquely traveling scatter (shown dashed) misses it, and the contrast is improved. Due to the inverse square law, the increased distance causes (a) a small reduction in the intensity of the primary radiation which comes from the anode, some distance away, but (b) a large reduction in the intensity of the scattered radiation, since that comes from points within the patient, much nearer. Use of an air gap increases contrast but necessitates an increase in the kV or mAs, and also results in a magnified image.

◆ *A flat metal filter.* Such a filter, placed on the cassette, absorbs the softer and obliquely traveling scatter more than the harder direct rays. This is not very effective, and necessitates an increase in the mAs.

2.3 SECONDARY RADIATION GRIDS

2.3.1 Effect on scattered rays

Few of the scattered rays S can pass through the channels between the strips of lead and reach the film. Since most of them are traveling obliquely and are relatively soft, they will be largely absorbed by the strips of lead. This is shown in greater detail in Fig. 2.7, A being the lead strips and B the interspace material. It will be seen that the grid has only a small *angle of acceptance* θ within which scattered rays can reach a point on the film.

Grid ratio

The grid ratio is the depth of the interspace channel divided by the width of the interspace channel, and is typically 8:1. The larger the grid ratio, the smaller the angle of acceptance, the more efficient the grid is at absorbing scattered radiation, and the greater the contrast in the image.

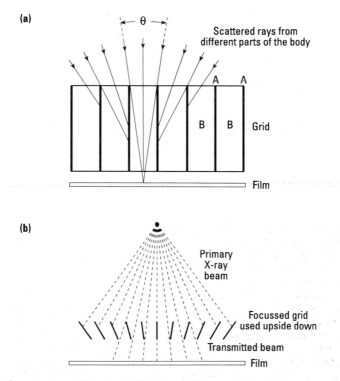

Fig. 2.7 (a) Construction of a grid. (b) Grid cut-off is caused by placing a focused grip upside down on the film.

With very large fields, especially at a high kV, more scatter is produced, and a *high-ratio grid* (12:1 or 16:1) is preferable. No grid would generally be used with thin parts of the body or with children or where there is an air gap.

Contrast improvement factor

The contrast improvement factor is defined as contrast with a grid divided by contrast without a grid. It lies typically between 3 and 5, depending on the grid ratio and the various factors affecting the relative amount of scatter produced.

Crossed grids

Unfortunately, scattered rays traveling obliquely to the primary beam but generally parallel to the lead strips can pass through the gaps. These rays can be absorbed by the use of crossed grids: two ordinary stationary grids superimposed with their grid lines at right angles. This is much more efficient than a single grid at removing scattered radiation, as the pathway for radiation is now a tunnel rather than a channel. However, crossed grids need a greater radiographic exposure and require very careful centering. If the grids are not at right angles, a coarse interference pattern (Moiré fringes) may be seen on the film. Grid cut-off can also be a problem (see Section 2.3.2).

2.3.2 Effect on direct rays

Focused and unfocused grids

In a focused grid the strips are tilted progressively from the center to the edges of the grid so that they all point toward the tube focus, as in Fig. 2.5. About 20% of the direct rays impinge on the edges of the lead strips and are attenuated. The rest pass through the gaps between the lead strips.

Grid cut-off

Within certain tolerances (a) the grid must be used at a specified distance from the anode, (b) the tube must be accurately centered over the grid, and (c) the grid must not be tilted; otherwise cut-off of the primary rays will occur. With a linear (i.e. uncrossed) grid, the X-ray tube can be angled along the length of the grid without 'cutting off' the primary radiation. This can be useful for certain examinations. If the tube is angled the other way, or if a focused grid is accidentally placed the wrong way round or upside down on the film, the primary beam will be absorbed, leaving perhaps only one small central area of the film exposed. This is known as 'grid cut-off' (see Fig. 2.7b), and is more restrictive with high-ratio grids.

Unfocused grids, in which the strips are completely parallel, may be used at any focus distance but suffer severely from cut-off. The effect can be reduced by using a longer FFD or a grid with a lower grid ratio.

Stationary and moving grids

Grid lines (grid lattice) are shadows of the lead strips of a stationary grid superimposed on the radiological image. If the line density (number of grid lines per millimeter) is sufficiently high they may not be noticeable at the normal viewing distance but they nevertheless reduce the definition of fine detail.

A *moving grid* ('Bucky') has typically five lines per millimeter. During the exposure it moves for a short distance, perpendicular to the grid lines. It can move to and fro (reciprocating) or in a circular fashion (oscillating). Such movement blurs out the grid lines. It is important that the grid starts to move before the exposure starts, moves steadily during the exposure, and does not stop moving until after the exposure is over.

A *multiline grid* has seven or more lines per millimeter together with a high grid ratio, and can be used as a stationary grid without the lines being visible. It is used when a moving grid cannot be used, and, being thinner, incurs less dose to the patient.

Speed and selectivity

The two tasks of a grid – to transmit primary radiation and absorb scattered radiation – may be judged by its selectivity:

$$\frac{\text{fraction of primary radiation transmitted}}{\text{fraction of scattered radiation transmitted}}$$

Typical figures range from 6 to 12, depending on the grid ratio and tube kV.

The use of grids necessitates increased radiographic exposure for the same film density, because of the removal of some of the direct rays and most of the scatter. Speed or exposure factor is the ratio

$$\frac{\text{total incident radiation}}{\text{total emergent radiation}}$$

or, in practical terms,

$$\frac{\text{exposure necessary with a grid}}{\text{exposure necessary without a grid}}$$

and is typically 3–5, depending on the grid structure, patient thickness, etc. Using a grid and, consequently, an increased exposure obviously increases patient dose.

Moving slot

An alternative to a grid consists of two metal plates each with a slot, 5 mm wide, aligned with the beam in front of and behind the patient. They are arranged to move steadily across the field during the exposure. With only a slice of the patient being irradiated at any instant, little scatter is produced. An increase of exposure time is necessary, but this can be mitigated by employing several slits well spaced apart.

2.4 MAGNIFICATION AND DISTORTION

Some important aspects of a radiological image arise simply from the fact that *X-rays travel in straight lines*. Figure 2.8a shows how the image I of a structure S produced by a diverging X-ray beam is larger than the structure itself.

If the diagram is redrawn with larger or smaller values for F and h, it will be seen that magnification is reduced by using a longer FFD F or by decreasing the object–film distance h. (It will be shown in Section 2.5 that this also reduces the blurring B.) When positioning the patient, the film is therefore usually placed close to the structures of interest. If the tissues are compressed this will also reduce patient dose. On the other hand, advantage is taken of increased magnification in macroradiography (see Section 3.9).

The *magnification M* is equal to

$$\frac{\text{length of the image}}{\text{length of the structure}}$$

and is given by $F/(F-h)$ in Fig. 2.8a.

Distortion

This refers to a difference between the shape of a structure in the image and in the subject. It may be due to foreshortening of the shadow of a tilted

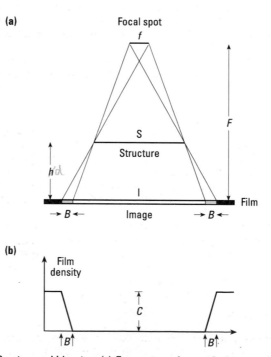

Fig. 2.8 Magnification and blurring. (a) Formation of magnified image. (b) A plot of film density along a line across the film.

object, e.g. a tilted circle projects as an ellipse. It may also be caused by differential magnification of the parts of a structure nearer to and farther away from the film–screen, an effect which is familiar to photographers. It can be reduced by using a longer FFD.

2.5 UNSHARPNESS AND BLURRING

Geometrical unsharpness

The image of a stationary structure produced by the beam from an ideal point source would be perfectly sharp. At the edge of the shadow, the intensity of X-rays would change suddenly from a high to a low value.

Figure 2.8a shows that, in the case of an effective focal spot f mm square, the intensity changes gradually over a distance B, variously called the penumbra, blurring or unsharpness.

If the diagram is redrawn with larger or smaller values for f, F and h, it will be seen that blurring is reduced by:

- using a smaller focal spot;
- decreasing the object–film distance; or
- using a longer FFD which also reduces magnification and distortion.

F is usually and conveniently 1 m, but it may be smaller in some techniques, such as fluoroscopy, while 2 m is used with a chest stand.

The geometrical blurring $B(g) = fh/F$ (approximately). If $f = 2$ mm, $F = 1$ m, and $h = 100$ mm, then $B(g) = 0.2$ mm. Usually the geometrical blurring is less than this as f and h are smaller.

Figure 2.8b plots the intensity of X-rays (or film density) along a line across the film. B is the geometrical blurring and C the contrast.

Movement unsharpness

One of the problems in radiography is the imaging of moving structures. If, during an exposure of duration t seconds, the structure moves parallel to the film with an average speed v, the edge of the shadow moves a distance slightly greater than vt. This produces movement blurring $B(m) = vt$ (approximately). If $v = 4$ mm s^{-1} and $t = 0.05$ s, then $B(m) = 0.2$ mm. (Movement strictly perpendicular to the film does not produce blurring.)

Movement blurring may be reduced to a satisfactory degree by immobilization and by using a sufficiently short exposure time, made possible by a rotating anode tube (see Section 2.7.2) and intensifying screens (see Section 3.4). It is, on the other hand, made use of in mechanical tomography (see Section 2.6).

Absorption unsharpness

A gradual change in absorption near the edge of a tapered or rounded structure, e.g. a blood vessel, produces absorption blurring. This is inherent in the objects being imaged, though the effect can sometimes be reduced by careful patient positioning.

In practice, all three types of unsharpness combine to limit the resolution achievable (see Section 3.6).

2.6 TOMOGRAPHY

So far we have considered conventional projection radiography, in which the shadows of structures farther from the film are superimposed on those closer to the film. This lack of depth resolution is overcome in biplane angiography by taking two crossed projections.

In tomography, only structures in a selected slice of the patient, parallel to the film, are imaged sharply. Those above and below are deliberately blurred so as to be unrecognizable. This blurring is produced by simultaneous movement, during the exposure, of two of the three following: tube, film, and patient.

In *linear tomography*, depicted in Fig. 2.9a, the tube T and cassette carrier C are linked by an extensible rod TC which is hinged about a fulcrum or pivot P which, in turn, is attached via a vertical arm to the table top. During the exposure, the cassette tray moves horizontally, for example from right to left, along rails under the couch top, while the tube stand moves along floor rails in the other direction, from left to right.

Figure 2.9b depicts two positions T_1 and T_2 of the focal spot and the corresponding positions of the film. It shows that the shadow of a structure P at the level of the pivot moves from P_1 to P_2 at the same speed as the cassette and therefore remains stationary on the film, producing a sharp

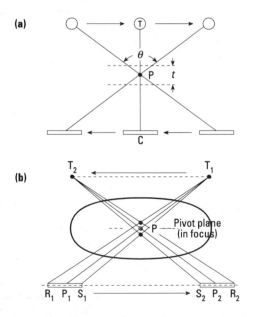

Fig. 2.9 Linear tomography (a) the thickness of cut t is related to swing angle θ. (b) Structures outside the focal plane are blurred.

image. This is true of any structure in the plane through P (sometimes called the 'focal plane'). However, the shadow of a structure R above the pivot moves further, from R_1 to R_2, sweeping across the film, and is blurred out. A structure S below the pivot is similarly blurred.

The farther the structure from the pivot plane, the greater the movement blurring. Structures lying within a slice of thickness t are sufficiently sharp to be recognizable, whereas those lying outside that slice are too blurred and of two low contrast (see below).

The *level of cut* is adjusted by raising or lowering the pivot. The *thickness of cut* (t in Fig. 2.9a) is controlled by adjusting the tomographic angle θ. The greater the angle of swing, the thinner the cut, because even structures vertically close to P are blurred. (On the other hand, if θ were zero, t would be very large, i.e. a conventional radiograph would result.) The thickness of cut also becomes smaller as the fulcrum (level of cut) is raised, as this increases the movement of the cassette and the tomographic effect. Decreasing the FFD has a similar effect.

Typically, in tomography θ is around 40° and t about 3 mm. Since such a thin slice of each structure is being imaged, and the shadows of off-focus anatomy are spread over the film, contrast is low, and a reasonably low kilovoltage must be used, consistent with penetrating the patient. The technique has been most useful when imaging structures of high inherent contrast, e.g. bony structures in the inner ear and iodine-filled vessels in pyelography. Since for much of the exposure the beam is passing obliquely through the patient, attenuation is higher and patient dose is greater than in conventional radiography. In *zonography*, θ is reduced to 5–10° and t is large enough to embrace the whole thickness of an organ such as the kidney.

If the tube and cassette movement run parallel to an elongated body structure, e.g. the femur, there will be comparatively little blurring of the long edges even when not in the pivot plane. To overcome this problem with linear tomography and increase blurring outside the pivot plane, other tomographic movements may be used:

- *circular movement*, which produces the tomographic effect in all directions;
- *elliptical movement*, similar to the above but more appropriate to the elongated human body; and
- *spiral* and *hypocycloidal movements*, on the principle that the more complex the movement the better!

Quality assurance

The performance of tomographic equipment can be checked for height of cut and slice thickness using commercial test tools. However, a simple test can be made by placing between the fulcrum and the table top a lead sheet with a hole 1 mm in diameter. Two exposures, one using a vertical beam and the other with the tomographic movement should produce an image of the swing (a straight line of uniform density for linear tomography) on which is superimposed a dense spot which should be at the center of the line.

If, alternatively, the hole is placed at the fulcrum, any elongation of the tomographic image of the hole indicates lack of coincidence between the movement of the tube and the film cassette. The angle of swing of the tube can be checked by placing a film cassette at a small angle to the vertical (narrowly collimated) beam, with the level of cut at the center of the film.

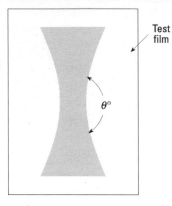

Fig. 2.10 Tomographic swing angle test image.

Figure 2.10 shows the resulting image, and the angle of rotation or swing is then given by $(180° - \theta)$, as shown.

2.7 LIMITATIONS OF THE X-RAY TUBE

There are two important limiting factors in imaging with X-rays: (a) the dose of radiation delivered to the patient, discussed earlier in this chapter, and (b) the heat which inevitably accompanies the production of X-rays. The latter affects the design of an X-ray tube and restricts the way in which it can be used. If this heat were to be allowed to accumulate in various parts of the X-ray tube, the consequent rise of temperature might cause damage and shorten or terminate the life of the tube.

In a radiographic exposure, excessive rise of target temperature, which might melt it, is avoided by spreading the heat over sufficiently large an area of the target and during sufficiently long an exposure time. On the other hand, to minimize focal spot and movement blurring, the focal area should be small and the exposure time short. A compromise between these opposing requirements is effected by two aspects of the design of an X-ray tube – the line focus and rotating anode.

2.7.1 Line focus

Left to themselves, the electrons emitted by the cathode, being mutually repellent, would spread and strike the target and produce X-rays over a large 'focal' area; thereby leading to blurred images. To obviate this, the helical filament is set in a rectangular slot in the cathode or focusing hood, which is connected to one end of the filament. This arrangement acts as an 'electron lens'. As a result, the electrons EE depicted in Fig. 2.11 are focused onto a small rectangular area AC on the target T. This is the *actual focal spot*, the area over which heat is produced and which determines the tube rating (see Section 2.7.3).

Because the target is tilted, the *effective focal spot* BC, seen from the center of the film, is foreshortened in one direction, and appears square. This ensures that the focal spot blurring is both small and the same

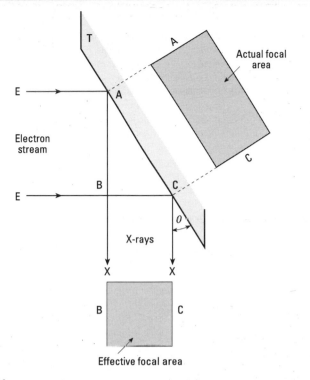

Fig. 2.11 Line focus.

whatever the orientation of a structure. However, the effective focal spot varies across the film. Seen from the cathode side of the film it is elongated in one direction, while from the anode side it is contracted in that direction.

The *target angle* θ is the angle between the central ray and the target face. The steeper the target angle (i.e. the smaller the target angle θ), the greater the foreshortening. Commonly, the target angle is 7 to 20°. If it is 17° and the effective focal spot is 1×1 mm, the actual focal spot must be 4×1 mm. Usually, an X-ray tube has two filaments and two focal spots of different sizes which are selected from the control panel. The smaller focal spot is selected for better resolution and the larger one for thicker parts of the body where a greater intensity of X-rays is needed (Table 2.1).

Table 2.1 Typical nominal[a] effective focal sixes (mm)

Macromammography	0.1
Mammography	0.3
Macroradiography	0.3
Radiography	0.6–1.2
Fluoroscopy	0.6

[a]The measured focal spot may be up to 50% larger than the manufacturer's specification.

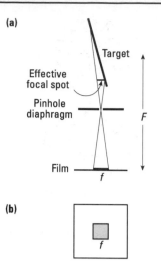

Fig. 2.12 Measurement of the effective focal spot with a pinhole camera. (a) Principle. (b) The resulting magnified image.

The steeper the target, the greater the foreshortening and the smaller the effective focal spot for the same actual focal spot and target heat rating. In other words, the steeper the target, the larger the actual focal spot and target heat rating for the same effective focal spot. On the other hand, as explained in Section 2.7.4, the steeper the target, the narrower the useful X-ray beam and the smaller the field covered. Thus, a steeper target may be more appropriate in mammography and also in cineradiography with a small field image intensifier than in general radiography using large films.

Measurement of the effective focal spot

There are two principal methods of measuring the effective focal spot.

A 'pinhole camera'. This consists of a hole drilled in a disk of heavy metal, such as gold, incorporated in a lead sheet. As shown in Fig. 2.12a, this is positioned between the tube and an X-ray film. The pinhole must be several times smaller than the focal spot. (Note that this diagram is not to scale: usually the FFD F is several hundred times greater than the effective focal spot f).

Although from each point on the target X-rays diverge in all directions, only one of them passes through the pinhole, and it produces a dot of blackening on the film. The resulting image (Fig. 2.12b) shows the shape of the focal spot and any lack of uniformity. It also reveals any extrafocal X-radiation, which is caused by electrons bouncing out of the focal area onto the surrounding target, and which would degrade the image. The pinhole is usually positioned much closer to the tube anode than to the cassette, so as to give a magnified image of the effective focal spot. Knowing the magnification enables the true size of the effective focal spot to be calculated.

(a)

(b)

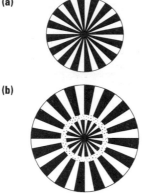

Fig. 2.13 Measurement of the effective focal spot with a 'star test' tool. (a) The 'star test' tool. (b) Image with a blurring diameter.

A 'star test' tool. A 'star test' tool or phantom comprises a number of tapered 'spokes' of lead mounted on a Perspex disk (Fig. 2.13a). This is mounted not in contact with the film but partway between it and the tube. Exposure produces a magnified and, in certain respects, an unsharp image of the star (Fig. 2.13b). In fact there is an obvious ring of blurring, the diameter of which is measured, and from this the effective focal spot size may be deduced. As will be seen in the diagram, outside this ring a sharp negative image is produced, as would be expected. Paradoxically, inside the ring there is a positive and reasonably sharp image of the spokes.

Blooming

This term refers to the increase in focal spot size which occurs when the tube is operated at a high milliamperage as the focusing is then less effective. It occurs particularly at low kV values and with small focal spots.

2.7.2 Rotating anode tube

Rotating the anode also increases the area over which the heat is produced and helps to dissipate it. The principle of a rotating anode is explained in Fig. 2.14. The simplest anode is a bevelled tungsten disk T which rotates during the exposure. The electron stream EE from the cathode is focused on the sloping edge of the disk.

The target is heated over the focal area (2, in Fig. 2.14b) and cools by conduction and radiation as it rotates round for further bombardment. In this way, hot metal is continually being replaced by cool metal and heat is spread over a focal track (1), say 200–300 mm long and 4 mm wide in the case of a 1 mm effective focal spot.

The anode assembly, seen in cross-section in Fig. 2.14a, consists of:

- An anode disk T, 7–10 cm or more in diameter, usually made of tungsten–rhenium alloy. This material has better thermal characteristics than pure tungsten and does not roughen with use as quickly.
- A thin molybdenum stem, M.

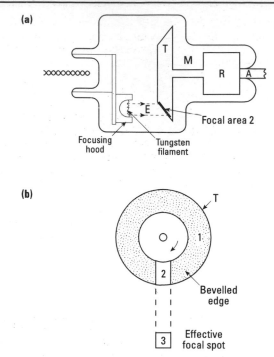

Fig. 2.14 Rotating anode tube. (a) Cross-sectional view. (b) Head-on view of the anode disk.

◆ A blackened copper rotor, R. This is part of the induction motor which rotates the target stem.
◆ Bearings, lubricated with a soft metal such as silver, which enable the rotor to rotate around the axle.
◆ An axle A, sealed into the glass envelope, which supports the target assembly.

The rotor rotates at about 3000 rpm, synchronously with the single-phase mains supply to the stator coil (the other half of the induction motor), mounted outside the glass envelope. High-speed anodes are energized with three-phase mains and rotate at about 9000 or 17 000 rpm.

How the anode cools

Heat produced on the focal track is conducted quickly into the anode disk and stored there temporarily, while being transferred by radiation to the insulating oil. The molybdenum stem is sufficiently long and narrow to control the amount of heat that is conducted to the rotor, so that it is not in danger of overheating and seizing up. Heat radiation is promoted by blackening the anode assembly. The rate of heat radiation increases as the anode gets hotter, being *proportional to the fourth power of the kelvin temperature*. Thus, a 40% increase in the output of X-rays and accompanying heat involves a rise of rather less than 10% in the kelvin temperature. Heat is next stored temporarily in the oil and is transferred by convection to the housing, from which it is lost by radiation and by fan-assisted convection through the surrounding air. High-powered tubes used in computed tomography and angiography may pump the oil through an external heat exchanger.

Other aspects of tube and generator design

The glass insert is immersed in oil, which convects heat away from the tube, the electrical insulating properties of which make for a more compact tube. The oil is contained in a metal housing which is earthed for electrical safety and lined with lead for radiation protection, except for a plastic window through which the useful X-ray beam emerges. The high tension and filament transformers are similarly contained in an oil-filled earthed metal tank and connected to the tube housing by a pair of highly insulated flexible cables, which also incorporate an earthed metal screen.

A low-powered dental X-ray tube is small and has a stationary anode: a tungsten target button embedded in a copper anode which serves as a temporary heat store.

2.7.3 Heat rating

The heat loading of an X-ray tube may be calculated in joules and is equal to $kV \times mAs$ for a constant potential (three phase) or $0.7 \times kV_p \times mAs$ for a pulsating single-phase generator.

Single radiographic exposure

In order to 'freeze' and display movement, individual exposures should be as short as the heating of the X-ray tube permits. Any combination of kV, milliamperage (mA), and exposure time used should be such that, at end of the exposure, the temperature of the anode does not exceed its safe value, i.e. there should be no risk of the target melting, vaporizing, emitting gas, or prematurely roughening. The *allowable mAs* at a particular kV increase as the exposure time is lengthened. Conversely, if the mAs needed to produce a satisfactory radiograph can be reduced, the exposure time can be made shorter.

The rating is usually stated as the *allowable mA*, and this:

- decreases as the exposure time is lengthened;
- decreases as the kV is increased, in inverse proportion;
- increases with the effective focal spot size and, for a given effective focal spot, is greater for smaller target angles;
- is greater for a rotating than a stationary anode;
- is greater for a 10 cm disk than a 7 cm disk;
- is greater for a high-speed anode because the heat is spread more evenly along the focal track;
- for exposures shorter than 1 s, is greater for a three-phase constant potential than for a single-phase pulsating potential – because the former produces heat more evenly throughout the exposure.

The foregoing information is stored on a microprocessor in the control circuit which prevents any exposure being made which would exceed the rating of the tube.

Repeated radiographic exposures

In order to display movement, as in angiography or cineradiography, a rapid series of exposures is made. Each exposure is sufficiently short to freeze movement, and each must be within the rating of the focal area. As a result of the repeated exposures, heat accumulates in the anode assembly and the oil. Neither of these can be allowed to exceed its maximum safe temperature. The rapidity with which a series of such exposures can be made depends on the maximum amount of heat that can be temporarily stored in the tube housing as a whole and the anode in particular; and on the rate at which they lose that heat by cooling processes. The heat storage capacity of the anode may be increased by soldering to the back of the tungsten plate a disk of molybdenum and/or solid graphite (both of which have a higher heat capacity per unit mass than tungsten).

When the kV, mA, and exposure time for each exposure and number of exposures required per second have been set, a microprocessor in the control circuit calculates the maximum total number of exposures allowed. If the anode heat capacity (typically 0.2 MJ) has been reached, it will need at least 15 min to cool down completely; but the entire assembly (typical heat capacity 1.0 MJ) may need an hour.

Continuous operation: fluoroscopy

If heat is produced on the focus continuously over a long period it must be removed at the same rate from the housing, if it is not to accumulate unsafely in the oil. The rating depends only on the cooling rate of the tube housing (and whether or not the fan is on) and not at all on the focal spot size or the type of generator. During fluoroscopy the anode may be stationary or else rotating at reduced speed, to reduce bearing wear.

Other ratings

There is a maximum kV which may be applied, depending on the insulation of the tube, cables, etc. There is a maximum mA that can be drawn without having to heat the filament to too high a temperature. The maximum mA is smaller at a low kV than at a high kV (due to what is called the 'space charge effect').

2.7.4 Uniformity of the X-ray beam

An X-ray tube emits some X-rays in every direction, necessitating lead shielding inside the tube housing to protect the patient and staff from unnecessary exposure. The useful beam is taken off where it is most intense, in a direction perpendicular to the electron stream. The central ray (B in Fig. 2.15) emerges at right angles to the tube axis from the center of the focal spot. It is usually pointed toward the center of the area of interest in the body.

Toward the anode edge A of the field the beam would be cut off by the face of the target. The beam could extend further in the cathode direction but is deliberately cut off at C by the edge of a circular aperture in the lead shield. Thus, the X-ray field is made symmetrical around the central ray B, and A and C are the limits of the useful beam.

In fact the useful beam is narrower than suggested because of the *heel effect*. As indicated in Fig. 2.15, most of the electrons penetrate a few

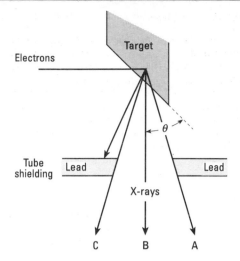

Fig. 2.15 Heel effect.

micrometers into the target before being stopped by a nucleus. On their way out, the X-rays produced are attenuated and filtered by the target material. It will be seen that X-rays traveling toward the anode edge of the field have more target material to cross and so are attenuated more than those traveling toward the cathode edge. The intensity of the beam decreases across the field from B to A. (Less importantly, the half-value layer (HVL) increases because of the filtration effect.) The steeper the target, the greater the heel effect. The longer the FFD, the less the heel effect with a given film size.

The heel effect, being gradual, is generally not noticeable even on the largest film. Where the patient's thickness varies considerably across the field, advantage may be taken of the heel effect by positioning the patient with the thicker or denser part toward the cathode of the tube where the exit beam is more intense (see, for example, mammography, Section 3.10).

The target surface roughens progressively during the life of an X-ray tube due to bombardment by the electrons. As a result, X-rays produced in the 'valleys' have to penetrate the 'hills' of tungsten, and this both reduces the output of X-rays and increases the heel effect. Overloading of the tube accelerates roughening and its adverse effects.

The intensity of the beam decreases somewhat either side of the central ray, in a direction perpendicular to AC (i.e. parallel to the tube axis), due to the inverse square law, the X-rays at the edges having farther to travel.

We have seen that two of the limiting factors in X-ray imaging are the amount of heat that is acceptable to the X-ray tube and the dose of radiation that is acceptable to the patient. A third limiting factor, the sensitivity and performance of the film–screen or other recording media will be the subject of the next two chapters.

2.7.5 Quality assurance of exposure parameters

Each X-ray tube and generator is produced to a certain specification and should be checked for compliance at installation. As exposure parameters such as the kV and mAs, and tube parameters such as the focal spot and filtration, can change with time, they need to be checked periodically. Each department will have protocols to follow, including the acceptable tolerances for each parameter, to preserve the quality assurance of the entire imaging system. This section highlights some of the tests which are performed. More details are given in Section 3.8.

Focal spot and filtration

At installation, the focal spot should be measured (see Section 2.7.1) and the total filtration checked. In Section 1.9, the effects of filtration were discussed, and in Section 1.4 the measurement of the HVL was discussed. If the HVL is measured carefully and the kV across the tube during the measurement is accurately known (see below), the total filtration can be deduced from a set of published graphs.

Kilovoltage and output

The kV can either be measured *directly* (and invasively) by using an instrument called a potential divider applied across the high tension leads, or *indirectly* (and noninvasively) by a penetrameter method. Usually, a calibrated electronic penetrameter is placed in the beam, and the instrument compares the differentially filtered response of detectors contained within it. This is analogous to comparing the first and second HVL to give an estimate of penetrating power, and it produces an equivalent kV.

The output of the tube can be measured using a dosemeter, often an ionization chamber. For a constant mAs, the output is a function of kV^x, where x is about 2, as mentioned in Section 1.9. For a constant kV, the output is a linear function of mA and exposure time, and, if the time is measured using an appropriate instrument, any discrepancy in the output curves can be attributed to malfunctions in either kV, mA, or exposure time.

Field definition and uniformity

The size of the X-ray field is delineated using lead diaphragms; for an overcouch tube there will be a light beam incorporated. Regular checks should be made to ensure that the light beam and field outline match and that the center of the field, on the cross wires of the light beam diaphragm, coincides with the center of the X-ray field.

In Section 2.7.4 the heel effect and field nonuniformity were discussed. The extent of this can be measured by exposing a large, plain film and measuring the density differences across the field.

VIVA QUESTIONS

1. Explain the term 'rating of an X-ray tube'.

2. What is the 'heel effect'?

3. What are the differences between the primary and secondary X-ray beams?

4. What affects the scattering of X-rays?

5. Draw a rotating anode tube.

6. How is heat dissipated from the anode?

7. What types of grid are there? Explain their uses.

8. In what types of radiography is an air gap used and why?

9. What is meant by the 'focal spot' and how can it be measured?

10. What is the principle of tomography?

11. What determines the thickness and level of a conventional tomographic slice?

12. What are the factors affecting radiographic contrast?

13. What is the relationship of patient absorbed dose to the kV and mA?

14. What are the causes of scatter?

15. How can scatter be reduced?

16. What are the causes of blurring seen on a radiograph?

17. What types of blurring or unsharpness occur? How can they be minimized?

18. What measurements can be made to ensure that the X-ray tube functions as specified?

3

RADIOGRAPHY WITH FILMS AND SCREENS

An X-ray cassette is a flat, light-tight box with spring clips and an internal pressure pad designed to keep its contents (usually a film between a pair of screens) in close contact. The front of the cassette, nearer to the tube, is made of aluminum ($Z = 13$) or, better, carbon fiber ($Z = 6$), in order to minimize the attenuation of the beam and so reduce the patient exposure required. Carbon fiber components (in the cassette, grid, or table top) are particularly effective at the lower kilovoltages (kV) values used in mammography, orthopedics, and angiography, compared with the higher voltages used in, say, barium studies. The cassette back usually incorporates a thin lead sheet to absorb the remnant radiation which would otherwise be back scattered, irradiating the patient unnecessarily and re-irradiating the screens, so degrading the image.

3.1 INTENSIFYING SCREENS

An intensifying screen consists of a polyester base (typically 0.25 mm thick) on which is coated a dense layer (0.1–0.5 mm thick) of fine phosphor crystals (3–10 μm in size) bound by a transparent resin. The crystals absorb X-rays and emit light of intensity proportional to the intensity of the X-rays. The screen faithfully converts the pattern of X-rays into one of light, which is then recorded by the film. The most frequently used phosphors are (a) calcium tungstate and (b) various rare earths – lanthanum oxybromide, lanthanum oxysulfide, and gadolinium oxysulfide (barium lead sulfate, barium fluorochloride, and yttrium oxysulfide have also been used).

To maximize the absorption of X-rays, the phosphor should have a sufficiently high atomic number. In this respect the absorption edge of

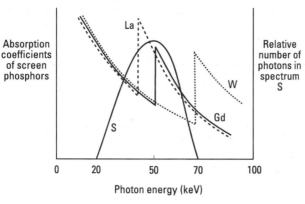

Absorption coefficients of screen phosphors

Relative number of photons in spectrum S

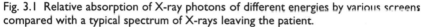

Photon energy (keV)

Fig. 3.1 Relative absorption of X-ray photons of different energies by various screens compared with a typical spectrum of X-rays leaving the patient.

tungsten (W, 70 keV) is less favorably placed in relation to the X-ray spectrum than those of gadolinium (Gd, 50 keV) or lanthanum (La, 39 keV). This is shown in Fig. 3.1, in which a typical spectrum S of X-rays generated at 70 kV reaching the film is superimposed on graphs showing the relative attenuation of screens incorporating salts of those elements. Rare earth screens are also more efficient than tungstate in converting absorbed X-ray energy into emitted light.

Both these factors make rare earth screens more sensitive ('faster') than calcium tungstate screens. They require a smaller exposure and deliver a patient dose 2–3 times lower, while producing images of the same quality. They may allow the use of a lower kV.

Matching film and phosphor

The intensity of light emitted by a screen depends on the phosphor, but its color depends on a small amount of an activator. The spectral sensitivity of the film should match the spectral emission of the screen. Thus, calcium tungstate, which emits a continuous spectrum of violet and blue light, and lanthanum oxybromide activated with the rare earth terbium, which emits a line spectrum of blue light, can be used with ordinary X-ray film, which is sensitive only to ultraviolet and blue light. An amber safelight can be used in the darkroom. Gadolinium and lanthanum oxysulfides activated with terbium emit a line spectrum of green light, and can only be used with an orthochromatic film, the sensitivity of which has been extended to include green light by coating the crystals with dyes. A red safelight is necessary.

3.2 FILMS

A film consists of a polyester base (typically 0.2 mm thick) on which is coated a thin photographic emulsion (10 μm thick). The emulsion is a suspension in gelatine of fine silver halide (iodobromide: 90% bromide, 10% iodide) crystals, each about 1 μm in size and containing a million or more silver atoms. Both films and screens have a very thin transparent antistatic supercoat to protect against abrasion, and are designed not to curl. A photographic emulsion is sensitive to X-rays, and ultraviolet and visible light. It is also affected by mechanical pressure and creasing, by static electricity, and by chemical liquids and vapors, all of which have implications for storage and handling.

Exposure to light

Two features of the silver iodobromide crystal account for the photographic process. The small proportion of iodide ions distort the lattice, which allows some of the silver ions to move through the lattice. The silver halide crystals are manufactured to possess sensitivity specks on their surfaces.

When a crystal absorbs a light photon, an electron may be liberated which migrates to the sensitivity speck, where its potential energy will be lowest. When a hundred or so photons have been absorbed by a crystal, enough electrons have accumulated at the sensitivity speck to attract mobile silver ions within the crystal to join them and be neutralized. They form a submicroscopic speck of silver metal, that is, a latent image in the film, awaiting development.

An X-ray film is usually double coated with an emulsion on each side of the base, and is used with a pair of screens. Each emulsion is in contact with the phosphor coating of an intensifying screen. About a third of the X-radiation falling on the front screen (nearer the patient) is absorbed and about half the light so produced travels forward and exposes the nearer (front) emulsion. About a half of the X-radiation transmitted by the front screen is absorbed by the rear screen, and of the light so produced, that which travels backward, exposes the rear-facing emulsion.

Processing

The invisible pattern of latent images is made visible by processing. The film is processed in three stages:

(1) The film is first *developed* by immersion in an alkaline solution of a reducing agent (an electron donor) which is able to enter the crystal at the site of the latent image. It proceeds to reduce the positive silver ions to silver atoms, and the latent image grows into a grain of metallic silver.

The unexposed crystals, which carry no latent images, are unaffected by the developer. The layer of bromine ions which form the surface of the crystal repel electron donor (developer) molecules and allow their entry only at the latent images where the ion barrier is breached.

In time, the developer would attack unexposed crystals. To inhibit this and so reduce fog, potassium bromide (restrainer) is incorporated in the initial charge of developer (but not in the replenisher since the reduction of silver itself liberates bromine ions into the developer). At this stage the film is wholly opaque.

(2) The film is now *fixed* by an acid solution of thiosulfate ('hypo'), which dissolves out the unaffected silver ions so that the image is stable and unaffected further by light. Incomplete fixation would leave the radiograph 'milky'.

(3) After each of stages (1) and (2) the film is *washed* in water, and finally it is dried by hot air. The result of inadequate washing would be for any retained hypo to turn brown/yellow.

Automatic processors use a roller feed system to transport the film through different solutions. Processor performance is maintained through a comprehensive quality assurance program, described in Section 3.3. Details of silver recovery from fixer solution and old films are given in Section 3.12.

Density

The film now carries a pattern of silver grains corresponding to the pattern of X-rays leaving the patient. The image is viewed by transmitted light on an illuminator or light-box of uniform brightness. It is a negative image: where the X-rays have been most intense, the film is darkest, and vice versa.

The grains of silver scatter and absorb the light as it passes through the processed emulsion. The optical density (D) of blackening of an area of the film depends upon the number of silver grains per unit area. It is found by measuring the ratio of the intensities of the incident and transmitted light using a densitometer:

$$D = \log_{10}(\text{incident light/transmitted light})$$

(The logarithm is used because the eye responds logarithmically to the brightness of light.)
For example,

if 1/100 of the light is transmitted	$D = 2.0$
if 1/10 of the light is transmitted	$D = 1.0$
if 1/2 of the light is transmitted	$D = 0.3$
if all the light is transmitted	$D = 0$

Densities are additive: if the front and rear emulsions each have a density of 1.0, the film has a total density of 2.0. The density of the area of interest on a properly exposed film averages 1.0; of the lung field in a chest film 2.0; while viewing an area of density of 3.0 needs a bright lamp.

3.3 CHARACTERISTIC CURVE

The response of a film and screen combination to X-rays is investigated by exposing different parts of it to different relative amounts (E) of X-rays and measuring their consequent densities (D).

The characteristic curve, drawn in Fig. 3.2, is the graph of D plotted against E on a logarithmic scale. E is properly the air kerma (in milligrays) but it is often called, loosely, 'exposure'. A logarithmic scale is used for E to match the exponential attenuation of X-rays in tissue. There are two important parts of the characteristic curve (indicated by the corresponding letters in Fig. 3.2):

(a) The *region of correct exposure* is the (nearly) straight-line portion, where the slope or gradient is steepest. The densities within the area of diagnostic interest should lie within this range.
(b) The *toe*, where the slope is shallow.

Other features are:

(c) the *shoulder*, where the slope is again shallow, and
(d) *saturation* density, in both of which the film is too dark to be readable on an ordinary illuminator;

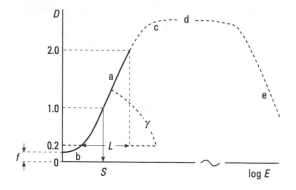

Fig. 3.2 Characteristic curve of a photographic film.

(e) *reversal* or solarization, which occurs when the exposure is sufficiently large – further increase causes a reduction in density, producing a positive image (this feature is exploited in reversal film, used for film copying, where direct exposure to mainly ultraviolet light is used to produce the copy).

Four properties of the film-screen combination can be derived from the characteristic curve:

(1) *Fog level.* This is shown as f in Fig. 3.2. It is the density of processed but unexposed film ($E = 0$). Fog reduces the contrast of the image and should be as low as possible. Inherent fog has typically $D = 0.12$ and is due, about equally, to (a) some of the silver bromide crystals having acquired latent images during manufacture and (b) the film base absorbing light when viewed. Additional fog may arise during storage (particularly if the temperature and humidity are too high or if the film is old) and from accidental exposure to X-rays. Fogging from light exposure produces a black pattern on the film.

(2) *Speed.* This is the reciprocal of the air kerma (S in Fig. 3.2) needed to produce $D = 1$, which is the average density of a properly exposed radiograph. In Fig. 3.3, film-screen A has a higher speed (is faster) than B. The speed of a film increases with the average grain size. Modern emulsions with flat crystals, aligned to face the X-ray beam, have a higher speed than those with rounder ones. Speed also depends on the photon energy of the X-rays (see also Section 6.9.1), being greatest at 30–40 keV.

The relative speed of two films or film-screen combinations is the ratio

$$\frac{\text{exposure needed to produce } D = 1 \text{ on one film}}{\text{exposure needed to produce } D = 1 \text{ on the other}}$$

It is shown as I in Fig. 3.3.

(3) *Gamma* (γ). This is also shown in Fig. 3.2. It is the slope of the straight-line portion of the characteristic curve. In Fig. 3.3, film-screen A has a higher γ (has a steeper slope, is more 'contrasty') than B.

In fact, the region of correct exposure is not quite straight. The slope

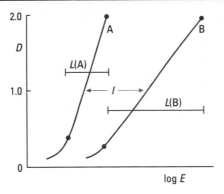

Fig. 3.3 Characteristic curves of two films or film-screen combinations.

increases as exposure and density are increased and γ generally refers to the average slope between densities 0.25 and 2.0 or 2.25.

The γ-value of a film depends on the *range* of crystal sizes (not their average size). The more uniform the crystals, the higher is γ, for the following reason. If all the crystals in an emulsion were of the same size, they would all acquire latent images at the same value of E, and the characteristic curve would be vertical, with a very high value of γ. Because they have a range of sizes, the smaller ones need a larger E than the bigger ones, accounting for the slope of the curve.

(4) *Film latitude or dynamic range.* This is shown as L in Fig. 3.2. It is the range of air kerma E which will produce densities D lying in the *useful density range* between (a) 0.25, below which the gradient is too low and (b) 2.0, above which the film is too dark for details to be seen using a normal illuminator. Typically the dynamic range is 40:1.

Figure 3.3 shows that γ *and latitude are inversely related*. It compares the characteristic curves of two film-screen combinations, A and B. A has the steeper slope and higher γ. It also has the narrower latitude $L(A)$. B, with lower γ, has the wider latitude $L(B)$. Typically, a wide latitude is needed in chest radiography and a high γ in mammography.

Exposure latitude

This refers to the range of exposure factors (kV and millampere-seconds (mAs)) which will give a correctly exposed image of a given subject. If the exposure latitude is too small, misjudgement of the machine settings appropriate to individual patients will necessitate repeating radiographs and incurring higher patient dose.

When a given subject is radiographed with a certain kV and mAs, the X-rays emerging from different parts of the region of interest cover a range of air kerma – from high values E_2, where the tissues are less attenuating (e.g. lung fields in a chest radiograph), to low values E_1, where they are more attenuating (e.g. diaphragm and mediastinum). This range of air kerma has to be faithfully captured on the film.

In Fig. 3.4a this range of air kerma E_1 to E_2 happens to fit *exactly* within the latitude of the film–screen. The film is correctly exposed but the

63

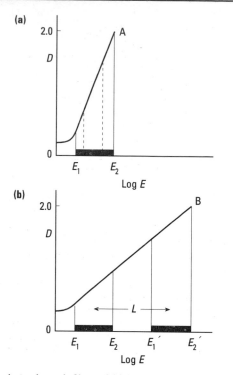

Fig. 3.4 Exposure latitude with films of (a) high and (b) low gamma.

operator has no latitude of exposure. If the mAs were reduced, it would shift the range of air kerma to the left and partially into the toe of the curve. The corresponding part of the image would have inadequate contrast. If the mAs were increased, it would shift the range of air kerma to the right, and part of the image would be too dense for contrasts to be seen.

In Fig. 3.4b, with a film–screen of lower γ the same range of air kerma covers only part of the wide film latitude. The mAs can be varied within the range L, while still producing a correctly exposed film, and this is called the *latitude of exposure*.

Returning to film-screen A in Fig. 3.4a, if a higher kV is used and the mAs reduced in compensation, the subject contrast is reduced. The range of air kerma within the image shrinks, as indicated by the dashed lines in Fig. 3.4a. There is now some latitude of exposure.

The exposure latitude therefore depends on both the film-screen latitude or γ and the range of kerma values being imaged, i.e. on the subject contrast. The latter in turn depends on the tissue densities, atomic numbers, and thicknesses of the structures in the beam and the tube kV employed. The exposure latitude for a particular radiograph of a patient can be increased by using a higher kV or a film of lower γ.

Effect of developing conditions

Increasing the developer temperature will increase the rate of chemical reaction and so cause an increase of speed but also of fog level. It also

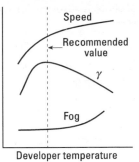

Fig. 3.5 Effect of developing conditions on speed, γ, and fog level.

causes γ to increase initially; but, above the temperature recommended by the manufacturer of the film, the increase in fog level will *reduce* the average γ (Fig. 3.5). Increasing developer concentration or developing time will have similar effects.

Developing conditions are optimized to give maximum γ and minimal fog. In an automatic processor, the *temperature* is controlled thermostatically, *time* by roller speed, and *concentration* by the speed of the developer replenisher pump, which in turn is controlled by the area of film being processed. As the concentration and temperature of the developer have a significant effect on speed, contrast, and fog, they must be controlled rigorously.

Quality assurance

Quality assurance of a processing unit is carried out to avoid the additional patient dose and waste of time and materials from having to repeat incorrectly processed films. It involves measuring the density, after processing, of at least three steps on a film on which a step-wedge image has been pre-exposed with light. For this, a device called a sensitometer is used. The first step (zero exposure) monitors *fog level*; the second ($D \approx 1$) monitors *speed*, and the difference between the second and third ($D \approx 2$) monitors γ. These densities are plotted daily, and a 10–15% variation in them is acceptable. Automatic readers are available which measure up to 20 steps and can produce a complete characteristic curve. They plot the variability on a day-to-day basis of the three basic quality assurance parameters, and indicate when and what remedial action should be taken.

3.4 USE OF SCREENS

Film exposed directly to X-rays

Direct exposure to X-rays of a film without screens produces a particularly sharp image, and is used in thin parts and where fine detail is required, e.g. teeth and bone fractures of the extremities. Whereas it requires some tens of light photons to produce a single latent image, each and every X-ray photon absorbed produces a latent image. This is because each single

Table 3.1 Number of photons absorbed for each 100 X-ray photons incident on the film/screen

Film and screen		Film only
Absorbed by phosphor,	30	Absorbed by film, 2
Light photons produced,	18 000	—
Light photons reaching film,	9 000	—
Latent images produced,	90	Latent images produced, 2

Intensification factor of screens = 90/2 = 45.

photoelectron set moving liberates a large number of electrons in the crystal.

Film exposed with screens

A film exposed with screens is more sensitive than the same film exposed alone for two reasons: the screen phosphor layer, being thicker, is more effective than the film emulsion at absorbing X-rays, and each 'large' X-ray photon absorbed by the phosphor produces many hundreds of 'small' light photons. Illustrative figures are given in Table 3.1.

Accordingly, the use of screens reduces the air kerma or exposure necessary to produce a properly exposed film. It therefore reduces the dose to the patient. It also reduces the loading of the tube and generator, thus allowing the use of shorter exposure times, and, consequently, reducing movement blurring. It may, possibly, also allow the use of a smaller focal spot.

Suppose that the characteristic curves in Fig. 3.3 now refer to a film used with screens (A) and to the same film used without screens (B). They show that, as well as increasing speed, the *use of screens increases* γ (from about 2 to about 3).

Intensification factor

The intensification factor (IF) or 'speed' of a pair of screens measures the reduction in patient dose and tube loading when the screens are used. It is the ratio

$$\frac{\text{air kerma necessary to produce } D = 1 \text{ with film alone}}{\text{air kerma necessary to produce } D = 1 \text{ with film plus screens}}$$

and is represented by I in Fig. 3.3. Typical values are 30–100. Because the absorption edges occur at different energies in the atoms in the film and phosphor respectively, the IF increases when the kV is increased.

The IF may be increased by increasing the thickness or 'coating weight' of the phosphor and by using larger crystals. It may also be increased by the use of a white reflecting layer, e.g. titanium dioxide, between the base and phosphor to reflect light traveling backward into the forward direction. Furthermore, rare earth screens have a larger IF than tungstate when producing images of the same quality (see Sections 3.7 and 3.12).

Front and back screens

To equalize the densities of the two emulsions, the rear screen coating is sometimes thicker than that of the front screen since the back screen relies on X-rays which have not been absorbed by the front screen.

Reciprocity law

This states that the density of blackening of a film depends only on the quantity of radiation (or mAs) whatever the particular combination of intensity (milliamperage, mA) and exposure time. It holds only for X-rays, i.e. film exposed without screens. It does not hold for light; when film is exposed with screens, the blackening produced, by the same mAs, in very short or very long exposures is less than with a 1 s exposure. This effect, a consequence of the involved way in which latent images are formed, can usually be ignored in clinical practice, except perhaps with the longer exposures in mammography.

Afterglow

Afterglow or delayed fluorescence (see Section 1.7) is to be avoided in intensifying screens as the screen retains a 'memory' of an exposure, which can be superimposed on the image of a subsequent exposure. More importantly, it is also to be avoided as 'lag' in the phosphor of an image intensifier (see Section 4.1) and 'dead time' in a gamma camera (see Section 5.4).

3.5 RADIOGRAPHIC CONTRAST

The contrast between adjacent areas of a film is the difference in their densities. In Fig. 2.4b the adjacent areas of the film–screen receive air kerma E_1 and E_2. Figure 3.4 shows that the same air kerma exposures E_1 and E_2 will produce a greater difference of density if film–screen A, which has a high γ, is used than they will if film–screen B, which has a low γ, is used. Thus, γ *amplifies contrast*:

radiographic contrast = film γ × subject contrast

Increasing γ increases the contrast. The factors which affect radiographic contrast are those which affect subject contrast (see Section 2.1) plus those which affect film γ (see Section 3.3). The greater the contrast, the less the exposure latitude. The foregoing refers to objective contrast. Subjective contrast, as seen by the eye, is affected by viewing conditions. It is reduced by glare from very bright areas of low attenuation, which should be masked off, and by too high a level of ambient lighting. (This refers equally to viewing a monitor screen.) Film viewing systems should be cleaned regularly and checked for adequacy of illumination.

3.6 SCREEN BLURRING

When a film is exposed without screens, a single X-ray produces in effect a point image. When screens are used, a single X-ray absorbed by a fluorescent crystal causes it to emit light in all directions. This is

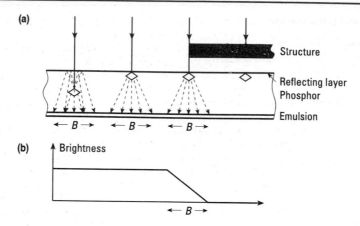

Fig. 3.6 Screen blurring. (a) Cross-section through film and screen. (b) A plot of brightness of phosphor image along a line across the screen.

illustrated in Fig. 3.6. Widely diverging light has far to travel in the phosphor coating, and is absorbed and scattered on the way and does not reach the film. Effectively, a cone of light is produced which is recorded as a small disk of blackening of diameter B. As the diagram shows, this light undercuts the edge of the shadow of a structure and produces blurring B which is typically 0.2 mm. Blurring can also be referred to as unsharpness U, or loss of resolution (see Section 2.5).

The thicker the screen coating or the larger the fluorescent crystals, the greater the blurring. Blurring can be reduced by (a) using thinner screens and finer crystals, (b) replacing the white reflecting layer by a black absorbing layer, and (c) incorporating dyes or pigments in the binder which further absorb the diverging light and reduce the size of the cone. All these measures also reduce the speed of the screen. Conversely, any measure taken to increase the intensification factor of the screen increases the unsharpness of the image.

As with all forms of imaging, a compromise has to be struck between speed or sensitivity and sharpness or definition. Screens are made to have either a high speed (fast screens, IF = 100) but larger blurring or a high definition but slower speed (detail screens, IF = 35). In addition, there are screens which compromise between speed and definition (par speed screens, IF = 50). Ultrafast screens may be used to reduce the patient dose from repeated exposures.

Rare earth screens are more effective than tungstate screens both at absorbing X-rays and converting the absorbed energy into light. They can either have a higher speed for the same resolution; or be made thinner and give sharper images for the same speed.

If there is poor *film–screen contact*, the disk of blackening produced by the cone of light is enlarged and the screen blurring increased. Poor contact, which may for example be due to a warped cassette or damaged hinges, appears as a region of reduced sharpness and contrast. This can be checked by radiographing a perforated metal sheet placed on top of the cassette; the image is darker and the pattern of holes indistinct where there is poor contact. Cassettes should also be tested for light leakage, which produces fogging around the edge of the film.

Parallax is another, less important, cause of blurring. Due to the diverging nature of the X-ray beam, the image on the rear emulsion is slightly larger than the front image, and, when viewed, this makes the edges of shadows less sharp. The effect is not noticeable except when the film is viewed wet and swollen or when the film is tilted relative to the central ray.

Another contribution to blurring is *crossover*, in which diverging light from the front screen reaches the rear emulsion and vice versa. It depends on the thickness of the film base and can account for 25% of the blackening.

In the newer *tabular* or 'T' grain film emulsions, the crystals are thin and flat with their surfaces aligned parallel to the film base to face the X-ray beam and will absorb light more efficiently. This reduces crossover, particularly if the base has been coated on both sides with light-absorbing dye. Completely isolating the two emulsions in this way has also led to the development of *asymmetric emulsion* films. A high-definition front screen is in contact with a high-γ emulsion, and a rear fast screen is in contact with a wide-latitude emulsion. The rear combination may be six times faster than the front. The combination can simultaneously image the sharp high-contrast structures in the lung and the denser structures of the mediastinum.

Single screens and single-coated films are used when definition is of prime importance, e.g. in mammography and bone detail radiography, and a reduction in speed can be tolerated. A back screen is used because, unlike a front screen, it produces most of its light nearest to the film.

Other uses of single-coated film

Ordinary photography uses single coated films with $\gamma = 1$. Single-coated films are used to record an image from cathode ray screens, e.g. in nuclear medicine and digital imaging; and in cineradiography or spot filming with an image intensifier (see Section 4.1.3). They are also used when copying radiographs with reversal film (which has been pre-exposed to bring it into the solarization region). Such film should have $\gamma = -1$ in order to produce a faithful copy of the original. These films are all matched to the spectrum of light to which they will be exposed, and formulated for automatic processing.

Combination of blurrings

A radiographic image may suffer simultaneously from screen blurring $B(s)$, just described, geometrical or focal spot blurring $B(g)$, and movement blurring $B(m)$, described in Section 2.5. The total blurring $B(t)$ perceived is less than the sum of the individual blurrings. It is more nearly the square root of the sum of the squares of the individual blurrings:

$$B(t)^2 = B(g)^2 + B(m)^2 + B(s)^2$$

For example, if it so happens that $B(g)$, $B(m)$, and $B(s)$ are each 0.2 mm, the total blurring will be about 0.35 mm (and not 0.6 mm). Suppose that $B(s)$ is reduced to 0.1 mm by using (slower) detail screens. To compensate, it may be necessary to increase the exposure by doubling the exposure time, thus increasing $B(m)$ to 0.4 mm. $B(g)$ remains at 0.2 mm. The total blurring then works out at 0.45 mm.

The foregoing illustrates two points:

(1) the minimum total blurring occurs when the individual blurrings are equal, or nearly so, and then

(2) in practice, any measure which aims to reduce one of the blurrings generally necessitates an increase in one of the others and in the total blurring.

Radiological imaging systems in general are designed with point (1) in mind.

3.7 QUANTUM MOTTLE OR NOISE

When a film is exposed with fast screens to a uniform beam of X-rays it would be expected that the blackening would be perfectly uniform over the film. In fact the density is likely to vary a little from one small area to the next, giving a mottled appearance.

Only photons that are absorbed in the film-screen convey information. Suppose that, in a radiographic exposure, an average of M photons fall on each square millimeter of a screen *and are absorbed*. Due to the stochastic nature of X-ray attenuation processes, the actual number of photons absorbed varies from one square millimeter of the image (or 'pixel') to another. Figure 3.7 shows graphically the relative number (R) of such pixels which each absorb a given number (N) of photons. About two-thirds (68%) of all pixels absorb between ($M - \sqrt{M}$) and ($M + \sqrt{M}$) photons. Sixteen percent absorb more than ($M + \sqrt{M}$) and 16% absorb less than ($M - \sqrt{M}$). The fluctuation in the number of photons absorbed is taken to be the standard deviation $\sqrt{M}$ of the function illustrated.

This random pattern of photons, called the 'noise' or quantum mottle, is superimposed upon the 'signal', the pattern produced by the structures in

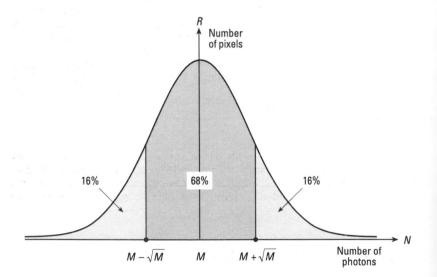

Fig. 3.7 Fluctuation in the number of X-ray photons absorbed in each square millimeter of a phosphor screen.

the patient. If the noise is too great it obscures the finer detail in the image. As will be further explained in Section 4.1.4, noise reduces the visibility of low-contrast shadows, particularly if they are small in area.

By the 'noise' in an image, we generally mean the relative noise, the ratio of the fluctuation $\sqrt{M}$ of photons absorbed to the average value M:

$$\text{relative noise} = \sqrt{M}/M = 1/\sqrt{M}$$

The larger the number of X-ray photons absorbed, the less noisy the image. Expressed in another way, the *signal-to-noise ratio* (SNR) is the ratio of the signal M to the noise $\sqrt{M}$:

$$\text{SNR} = M/\sqrt{M} = \sqrt{M}$$

The larger the number of X-ray photons absorbed, the greater is the SNR:

Number of events	Noise	SNR
100	10%	10:1
1000	3%	30:1
10 000	1%	100:1
100 000	0.3%	300:1

In a typical radiographic exposure M = 100 000 photons mm^{-2}, and the SNR = 300:1.

The SNR should be high to maximize information. If the SNR is low, the image appears 'noisy'. The use of screens increases noise. Remember that the aim is to produce a certain film density. A fast screen requires a lower X-ray dose or exposure (fewer photons mm^{-2}) and gives a worse SNR. A slow or detail screen requires a higher X-ray dose or exposure (more photons mm^{-2}) and gives a better SNR. For the same sharpness, a rare earth screen is faster than a tungstate screen and so produces more quantum mottle. This may, however, be outweighed by the reduced patient dose.

Similarly, using a higher kV involves fewer and higher-energy photons and so less dose to the patient but reduces the SNR. As a general rule, in all imaging systems, measures to reduce the effect of noise and increase the SNR will increase patient dose. For further details, see Section 3.12.

Other less important forms of noise

The fact that a screen is made of individual crystals may produce a small degree of *structure mottle*. The fact that a film image is made of individual grains may produce an even smaller degree of mottle or *'graininess'*. The latter mainly becomes evident when, as with cine film, the image must be magnified for viewing.

3.8 CHOICE OF EXPOSURE FACTORS

The controls of an X-ray set usually include kV and two out of the three factors: mA, exposure time, and mAs (Table 3.2). In making a particular

Table 3.2 Examples of exposure factors

Examination	Exposure factors
Barium meal (screening)	90 kV 0.5 mA (up to 5 mA if necessary)
Average adult chest X-ray	70 kV 10 mAs comprising a high mA (e.g. 300–500 mA) and a short exposure time of only a few milliseconds (e.g. 0.02 s)
Chest X-ray (high-kV technique)	120 kV 4–5 mAs composed similarly to the average adult chest X-ray above

radiological examination, when screens are used the film dose (see Section 2.1) is approximately proportional to $kV^4 \times mAs$, so that kV and mAs have to be considered together. As a rule of thumb, since 90^4 is twice 75^4, increasing the tube voltage by 15 kV allows the mAs to be halved when imaging a given subject.

Kilovoltage. In general, as high as possible a kV will be used so as to (a) increase the penetration of the beam and reduce patient dose, (b) increase the latitude of exposure and range of tissues displayed, and (c) reduce the mAs needed and thus allow shorter exposure times, within the rating of the tube; but (d) not so high a kV that insufficient contrast results in the area of diagnostic interest.

Milliampere-seconds. Having chosen the kV for a particular examination, this determines the required mAs, which is then subdivided into (a) as short as possible an exposure time (to arrest motion) and (b) a correspondingly high mA – just within the rating of the tube, as described in Section 2.7.3.

Exposure time. The necessary exposure time can be reduced by selecting (a) a higher kV and (b) a larger focal spot. However, as explained in Section 3.6, using a larger focal spot to reduce the exposure time may sometimes increase the overall blurring. Focal spot size, exposure time and screen speed should be chosen together, to give minimal total blurring, which occurs when the separate blurring components are approximately equal.

The necessary exposure time can also be reduced by using:

- a three-phase generator, rather than single phase;
- full-wave single-phase rather than self-rectification; and
- a higher speed and larger-diameter anode disk.

High-kilovoltage radiography

This is carried out at maximum kV (say, 150 V), the mAs being selected according to the thickness and nature of the part being radiographed. In consequence:

◆ subject contrast is low, which allows a wider range of tissue to be imaged on a film, making the choice of mAs less critical and possibly reducing the number of repeat exposures;
◆ skin dose is reduced;
◆ efficiency of X-ray production is high, thus reducing the heat loading and allowing very short exposure times;
◆ the amount of scattered radiation is relatively high, thus making grids less effective (the use of an air gap is generally preferred).

Automatic exposure control (AEC)

Having selected the kV, the exposure can be terminated automatically when exactly the right mAs has been delivered to expose the film correctly, irrespective of any misjudgement of the ideal kV (in respect of patient thickness, etc.) or of fluctuations in the mains supply.

The exposure is controlled automatically by placing a thin sensor on top of the cassette to measure the intensity of the X-rays. This may be either a flat parallel-plate ionization chamber (see Section 1.8) or a phosphor, which converts the X-rays to light, coupled to a photo-multiplier, which measures the light. Often three sensors are placed at different locations in the X-ray field, which allows control of the exposure to one region of interest or an average exposure over two or three areas. The radiologist's preference for 'light' or 'dark' films is accommodated by a sensitivity or density control.

The control device should not attenuate the beam very much, is generally larger than the cassette, and must not itself produce an image on the film. In some designs of sensor, this last requirement would not be met, and it must be placed behind the cassette, which should then not incorporate the usual heavy metal backing.

Quality assurance

Reject analysis of all films which are not of diagnostic value should identify which of positioning, patient movement, choice of exposure factors, equipment, or processing is at fault. Action can be taken accordingly. To avoid repeat films and unnecessary patient dose, the following parameters – which can vary with time – should be checked on each tube and generator after each service, at least, and whenever there appears to be a lack of consistency of exposure.

The actual tube kilovoltage should be within ±5% of the set value. It can be measured *directly* (and invasively) by applying an instrument called a potential divider across the high-tension leads. It can more easily be estimated *indirectly* (and noninvasively) by a penetrameter method. A typical kV check meter employs two copper absorbers of different thicknesses, beneath each of which is a photodiode. The unit is positioned in the middle of the X-ray field, some 50–75 cm from the tube. Attached to the tube is a 0.5 mm copper filter which transmits mainly X-rays near to the peak kiloelectronvolt value. Tube kV, mA, and exposure time are selected, and an exposure made. Each detector produces a different current, proportional to the X-ray intensity falling on it. The higher the tube kV, the smaller the ratio of the two currents. The current ratio is displayed, as the equivalent kV, on a digital read-out. The general nature of the waveform (pulsating or constant) can also be displayed. The kV is checked at several settings of the kV control. The kV meter itself needs to have the accuracy of its readings checked periodically at a national or secondary standards laboratory.

In the same meter, the current from a single diode may be:

◈ Displayed to monitor consistency of *X-ray output*. (For greater accuracy, the output may be measured with a dosemeter such as an ionization chamber. The measured values should increase linearly with mA and kV^x, where x is about 2 (see Section 1.9). Automatic exposure controls are similarly checked by measuring the radiation front and back of a water phantom with a dosemeter.)

◈ Used to start and stop a built-in digital timer to measure pulse length or check *timer* accuracy.

◈ Displayed on an external storage oscilloscope, showing the *waveform* more precisely, how quickly the X-rays switch on and off, and the exposure time.

The total *filtration* (which might have been disturbed during servicing) may be checked by measuring the kV (as above) and the half value layer (HVL) (see Section 1.4) and referring to a set of published graphs. Figure 1.13a shows the correct conditions for measuring the HVL. A narrow beam is used, collimated so as just to cover the ionization chamber detector. Scattered radiation is minimized if the aluminum absorbers are placed about half-way between tube anode and the detector. The *focal spot* may also be checked when a new tube is installed, as described in Section 2.7.1.

3.9 MACRORADIOGRAPHY

Where a magnified image is required, the anode–object distance is decreased relative to the object-film distance, which is increased. Figure 3.8

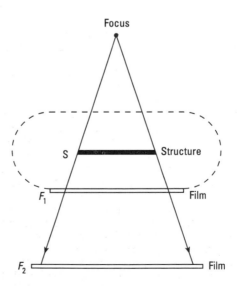

Fig. 3.8 Macroradiography.

shows that the image of a structure S is larger when the film F_2 is some distance from the patient than when it is at F_1, close to the patient. This has the following implications for technique:

◆ *Focal spot*. A very small focal spot must be used (e.g. 0.1 mm) otherwise geometric blurring would be unacceptable. As a result, the heat rating is reduced.

◆ *Exposure time*. Exposure times may have to be increased to several seconds, to keep within the rating of the focal spot and as a result increased movement blurring may result. *Immobilization* is therefore important.

◆ *Patient dose*. Patient dose is increased because of the increased exposure needed.

◆ *Contrast*. No grid is needed as the air gap reduces the scatter reaching the film. This helps to reduce the additional exposure needed.

◆ *Screen blurring*. Screen blurring is not magnified although the image of the structure is. In other words the relative effect of screen blurring is reduced. This means that fast screens may be used, which again helps to reduce the additional exposure needed.

◆ *Geometrical blurring*. Geometrical blurring is increased, relative to the size of the image.

◆ *Quantum mottle*. Quantum mottle is not increased, since the same number of X-ray photons are absorbed in the screen, for the same film blackening.

3.10 MAMMOGRAPHY

Mammography aims to demonstrate both microcalcifications as small as 100 µm in size of high inherent contrast and larger areas of tissue having much lower contrast, on the same film.

Contrast

The breast does not attenuate the beam greatly, allowing the use of the low kV that is needed to obtain sufficient photoelectric absorption in order to differentiate between normal and abnormal breast tissues. Ideally, monoenergetic X-rays of about 18–20 keV would produce optimal contrast and penetration in the case of a small breast.

This can be approximated by operating a tube having a beryllium window and a molybdenum target at 28 kV (constant potential) and using a 0.03 mm molybdenum filter which has an absorption edge at 20 keV. This transmits most of the characteristic radiation (17.9 and 19.5 keV) but removes most of the continuous spectrum. Figure 3.9 compares (A) the spectrum produced in this way by a molybdenum–molybdenum combination with (B) the spectrum that would be produced by operating a tube with a tungsten target at 30 kV and using a 0.5 mm Al filter.

With the thicker breast, higher-energy radiation is preferred. Better results, with a significant decrease in absorbed dose to the breast tissue, are obtained with a rhodium or a palladium filter, having absorption edges at 23 and 24 keV, respectively. Better still is a tube with a rhodium target, giving 20.2 and 22.7 keV characteristic rays, used with a rhodium filter.

The small focal spot and the inefficient production of X-rays consequent on the low kV and target atomic number incur problems of tube loading.

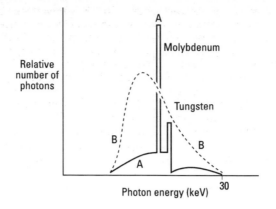

Fig. 3.9 X-ray spectra using a molybdenum target and filter (A) and a tungsten target with an aluminum filter (B).

Films with a value of γ of about 3 are used. Contrast is also improved (but the exposure and patient dose are increased) by the use of a grid or air gap. A very fine grid is the preferred option.

Image definition

Imaging microcalcifications is not easy. It is necessary to use a single coated film to avoid parallax and crossover, together with a single, rare earth, rear screen. A vacuum cassette improves the film–screen contact. A small focal spot (0.3 mm or less) must be used and, for magnification of suspected lesions (by factors of 1.5 or 2, using an air gap of 15–30 cm) 0.1 mm focal spots are used. On account of the small field of view, a 10° target can be used, or a 0° target with the tube tilted away from the chest wall. A metal (not glass) tube is often used; this has little extrafocal radiation.

Compression of the breast is vital for immobilization since, taking all the above factors into account, exposure times are relatively long. Compression is also used to reduce the object–film distance and so reduce geometric blurring; and to equalize tissue thickness. Even so, the narrow exposure latitude with high-γ film–screens make automatic exposure control, carefully controlled processing, and daily quality assurance checks desirable for consistent films and to avoid repeats.

Dose

The requirements of contrast and of sharpness or spatial resolution tend to increase patient dose. Careful attention to technique is therefore necessary since breast tissue is relatively sensitive to radiation. The beam is tightly collimated and the collimator is designed to protect the chest wall from irradiation, and the rest of the body is protected by absorbing the remnant radiation immediately behind the cassette.

Ironically, while the objective of mammography is the early detection of breast tumors, irradiation of breast tissue is itself carcinogenic. Typically the average dose to glandular tissue in the breast is 2 mGy per mammogram, which carries a risk of inducing fatal cancer of about 20/million at age 30–50 years and 10/million at age 50–65 years (see Section 6.3). This has implications for routine mammography of 'well women' outside recognized breast-screening programs.

Mammography equipment is subject to strict *quality assurance* procedures. The usual tube and generator tests are carried out, using special equipment for the low kV and filtration involved. In addition, image quality and patient dose are crucial factors. Collimation and field alignment are particularly important. A mammography phantom capable of producing an anthropomorphic image, in addition to quantifiable data (for contrast and resolution), is ideal for routine use. The mean glandular dose is also measured periodically, using a special thin-window ionization chamber and a standard Perspex mammographic phantom.

3.11 XERORADIOGRAPHY

Xeroradiography employs the same principle as a photocopier. Instead of a film and screen, the light-tight cassette contains a rigid aluminum sheet (A in Fig. 3.10) on which is coated a thin layer (S) of selenium. Before exposure to X-rays its surface is sprayed with a uniform positive charge, as indicated in Fig. 3.10a.

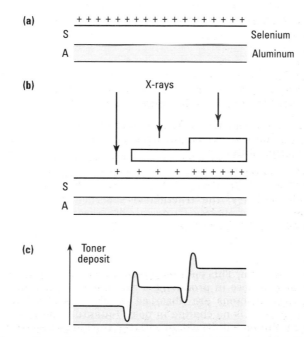

Fig. 3.10 Xeroradiography. (a) Cross section through charged selenium plate. (b) Exposure to X-rays with a step-wedge. (c) Plot of density of toner deposit along a line across the plate.

In the dark, this material is an insulator but, when exposed to X-rays (or light), electrons are liberated within the material, and these progressively discharge the positive surface charge. The charge remaining at any point on the surface is related to the exposure of X-rays it has received. Thus the X-ray pattern is converted into a pattern of positive charge. Figure 3.10b shows the distribution of charge left after radiographing a stepped structure.

Processing is rapid and 'dry'. The image is developed, in the dark, in a closed development chamber by an aerosol of fine particles of carbon or dark blue thermoplastic toner material. These are negatively charged and so are attracted to the remaining charge on the plate. The image is then transferred to a paper sheet which is heated to bond the toner particles permanently. The selenium plate is reused after cleaning and recharging.

Figure 3.10c shows the distribution of toner resulting from the exposure of Fig. 3.10b. More toner is accumulated for denser body structures, so the image produced is a reversal of a normal X-ray film. The image generally has a very low contrast as the density of the carbon deposit does not vary greatly over the image. However, the boundaries of structures are well delineated by 'edge enhancement'. Figure 3.10c shows that the toner piles up along one side of a boundary and is correspondingly depleted along the other side.

As a result, structures of about 1 mm in size stand out particularly well and show a much higher contrast than larger structures. For this reason xeroradiography has sometimes been used in mammography, in which case a tungsten anode gives better results than a molybdenum one. However, as it generally incurs a higher dose than with films and screens, it is no longer favored as an imaging technique.

3.12 APPENDIX

Intensifying screens: speed and noise (see Section 3.7)

The IF of a screen depends on the product of the following three factors (approximate values are given in brackets; rare earth screens are more effective than tungstate):

- *X-ray absorption*, the fraction of incident X-ray photons that are absorbed in the screen (tungstate 30%, rare earth 60%);
- *conversion efficiency*, the fraction of absorbed X-ray energy that is converted into light photons (tungstate 5%, rare earth 20%);
- *screen efficiency*, the proportion of the light produced in the screen that reaches the film (50%).

The IF can be increased by increasing X-ray absorption, for example by using a thicker screen. This enables a reduction in the necessary exposure, and so the patient dose in producing a satisfactory radiograph. The same number of X-ray photons are absorbed in the screen for the same film density and so there is no change in noise (quantum mottle) although the blurring or resolution will be worse with the thicker screen.

The IF can also be increased by increasing the conversion or screen efficiency. In each case this reduces the number of X-ray photons that need to be absorbed for the same film density. The exposure needed and the

Table 3.3 Summary of effects on image quality of increasing screen speed

Screen change	Noise	Resolution
X-ray absorption	Same	Same
Density	Same	Same
Screen thickness	Same	Worse
Conversion efficiency	Worse	Same
Screen efficiency	Worse	Worse

patient dose incurred when producing an acceptable film are again reduced, but the noise (quantum mottle) is increased. Increasing the screen efficiency, for example by using a reflecting layer, reduces resolution, but increasing conversion efficiency does not affect it.

Thus, *increasing conversion efficiency increases quantum noise but increasing screen thickness does not*; both increase the speed of a screen and reduce patient dose.

The effects of increasing the speed of a screen on image quality are summarized in Table 3.3.

Silver recovery

Silver is an expensive and relatively scarce material which also causes pollution if disposed of in the environment. As large amounts of silver are left behind in film processing, it is important to recover as much as possible for recycling. There are a number of ways to reclaim the silver:

- In the *electrolytic method*, 90–95% of the silver in fixer can be deposited on a rotating cathode. The fixer can be reused. To avoid sulfiding (formation of silver sulfide) the pH must be kept low.
- Silver can be recovered from fixer or wash water by *metallic displacement* with iron wool. Silver is precipitated as a sludge, and needs refining. The fixer cannot be reused.
- Silver may be recovered from *scrap film* by burning or by chemical treatment.

VIVA QUESTIONS

1. How is a cassette constructed?

2. Why are intensifying screens used, and how do they work?

3. What problems arise with poor film-screen contact?

4. What are the differences between calcium tungstate screens and rare earth screens?

5. How is a latent image produced?

6. What are the differences between single- and double-emulsion films and when are they used?

7. How does an automatic processor work? What quality assurance program should be followed?

8. What is meant by (a) the density, (b) the characteristic curve, (c) γ, (d) the speed, and (e) the latitude of a film?

9. Draw a plot of density D against exposure E of a film.

10. What does the term 'radiographic contrast' mean and what factors influence it?

11. What is quantum mottle and what affects it?

12. What physical features of the X-ray system are necessary to perform macroradiography?

13. Why is molybdenum used in mammography as a target and a filter?

14. Draw the spectra of X-ray tubes operated at 30 kV using tungsten and molybdenum as targets and, show their differences.

15. Explain briefly the processes involved in xeroradiography.

16. What are typical screening mA and kV values and how do they compare with the exposure for a chest radiograph?

17. What sorts of faults can be identified through film reject analysis and what steps can be taken to reduce the reject rate?

4

FLUOROSCOPY, DIGITAL IMAGING, AND COMPUTED TOMOGRAPHY

4.1 FLUOROSCOPY

In fluoroscopy, an instantaneous ('real time') and visible image is produced by a phosphor screen which converts the pattern of X-rays leaving the patient into a pattern of light. Since the intensity of light is proportional to the intensity of X-rays, it produces a faithful image, with $\gamma = 1$.

In the early days, *direct vision fluoroscopy* used a zinc sulfide screen, and the radiologist was protected from the primary beam by a sheet of lead glass. Even using a dose rate then considered acceptable for the patient, the brightness of the screen would be too low to stimulate, in the retina of the eye, the cones which are used in normal reading and when viewing films or a video screen (photopic vision). Although the sharpness and contrast of the image was nearly as good as on a film, the eye could not appreciate it. Relying as it did on rod (scotopic) vision, the visual acuity and the ability to perceive contrast were both only about 1/10 as good as in radiography. Even that was achieved only by screening in a rather dark room after 10–20 min of dark adaptation, wearing red goggles. All these problems, and particularly that of high dose to the patient, disappeared with the advent of the image intensifier, and indeed the use of direct-vision fluoroscopy is now banned.

4.1.1 The image intensifier

In the image intensifier, electrical energy is used to increase the brightness of the image, while maintaining its proportionality with the X-ray beam intensity.

As Fig. 4.1 shows, the evacuated glass envelope (1) contains an input screen, 230 mm or more in diameter. This incorporates a phosphor screen (2) 0.2 mm thick, coated on the inside of the glass, made of fine crystals of cesium iodide. The phosphor absorbs about 60% of the X-ray energy and converts the X-ray pattern into one of light. Coated over the phosphor screen is a cesium–antimony photoelectric screen or 'photocathode' (3) which converts the light pattern into one of electrons.

The light photons knock electrons out of the photocathode. The electrons are accelerated by 25–35 kV between the negative input and positive output screens. They are focused, to preserve the image, by one or more cylindrical electrodes (4) at intermediate potentials. These constitute an 'electron lens'. The metal housing provides some shielding against external magnetic fields as well as X-ray protection.

The accelerated electrons impinge on the smaller output screen. This is typically 25 mm in diameter, incorporates a phosphor screen (6) coated on the inside of the glass, and made of very fine crystals of zinc–cadmium

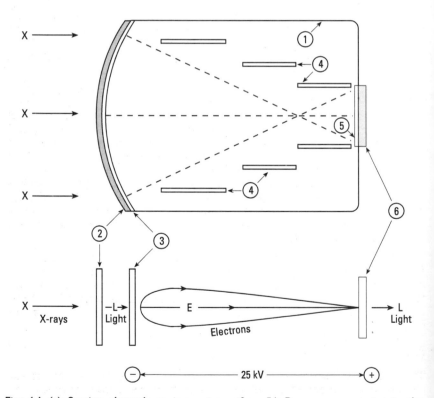

Fig. 4.1 (a) Section through an image intensifier. (b) Processes occurring in the intensifier.

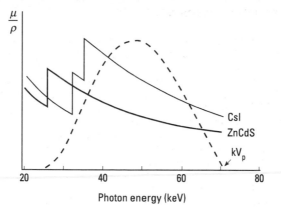

Fig. 4.2 Mass attenuation coefficient of cesium iodide (CsI) and zinc–cadmium sulfide (ZnCdS) versus photon energy with the X-ray spectrum superimposed.

sulfide, activated with silver. These convert the electron pattern back into one of light. The phosphor is covered with a thin aluminum film (5), through which the accelerated electrons penetrate.

Cesium iodide (compared to, say, zinc-cadmium sulfide) is preferred for the input phosphor because:

◆ Its absorption edges (at 33 and 36 keV) are favorably placed in relation to the effective energy of the X-ray spectrum. In Fig. 4.2, a typical spectrum of X-rays incident on an image intensifier is superimposed upon graphs of the attenuation coefficients of zinc–cadmium sulfide and cesium iodide versus photon energy. It shows that the greater part of the spectrum of X-rays leaving the patient lies on the high absorption side of the absorption edge of cesium iodide.

◆ Its fine needle-like crystals can be aligned with the X-rays and packed together closely so that they act as miniature light guides, thus reducing light spread. This increases the efficiency of the screen, which reduces patient dose and also allows a thinner screen, thus reducing screen unsharpness.

Light spread is not a problem with the output screen, for it need only be a few micrometers thick, since it has to absorb electrons, not X-rays. The aluminum foil prevents light from the output phosphor traveling backward to the input photoelectric screen and causing further emission of electrons and ultimately of light. Such optical feedback would reduce the image contrast.

Gain

The image is intensified, minified, and inverted by the action of the electron lens. For each X-ray photon absorbed by the input phosphor about 400 light photons are emitted, producing some 400 photoelectrons, which then cause the output phosphor to emit nearly 400 000 light photons.

Intensification can be measured in two ways:

◆ *Brightness gain* is the ratio

$$\frac{\text{brightness of the output phosphor}}{\text{brightness of the input phosphor}}$$

and is not directly measurable. The overall gain is typically 5000–10 000 and is the product of two factors:

(a) Flux gain (the increase in the number of light photons due to the acceleration and hence gain in energy of the electrons): 50–100 times.

(b) Minification gain, which is equal to the area of the input phosphor divided by the area of the output phosphor: about 100 times. Using a smaller output screen would make the image even brighter but also more grainy.

◆ *Conversion factor* is the ratio

$$\frac{\text{brightness or luminance of the output phosphor (candela/m}^2)}{\text{dose rate in air on the input surface of the intensifier (}\mu\text{Gy/s)}}$$

measured with a photometer and a dosemeter employing a flat circular ionization chamber, respectively. Typical figures are in the range 15–25, but it decreases with age and use.

Compared with the center of the image, the edges tend to be less bright, less sharp, and more distorted, due to difficulty in control of the peripheral electrons by the electron lens. The problem is partly met by curving the front face of the intensifier.

Dual- and triple-mode intensifiers

By changing the voltages of the intermediate electrodes, the electron crossover point can be moved nearer to the patient so that the intensifier operates in a magnification mode. The central part of the input image (160 or 110 mm in diameter) then fills the whole of the output phosphor. This magnifies the image and improves the sharpness or resolution but makes the image less bright, necessitating an increase in exposure factors. This increases the patient's skin dose, but the X-ray beam is automatically recollimated, so that the volume of tissue irradiated is reduced and so is the scatter, improving contrast.

Beam splitter

Figure 4.3a shows how light is collected from the output phosphor (2) by a lens (3) and then, at choice, either

◆ collected by the lens (4) and focused on the input screen (5) of a television (TV) camera, part of a closed-circuit TV system, or

◆ reflected (90%) by a 45° partial mirror (1) onto the lens (6) of either a camera loaded with cut film or a cine camera (7); the remaining 10% falls on the lens of the TV camera, allowing the image to be monitored during photography.

Alternatively, if film cameras are not to be used, the image intensifier can be coupled to the TV camera by fiber optics.

(a)

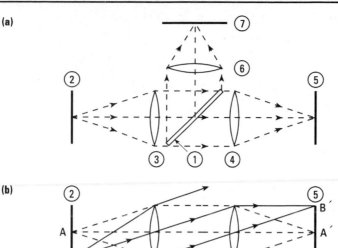

(b)

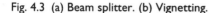

Fig. 4.3 (a) Beam splitter. (b) Vignetting.

Vignetting

The center of the final image is brighter than its edges. Figure 4.3b shows that all the light from the center A of the output phosphor (2) that is collected by the first lens (3) is collected and focused by the second lens (4) onto the image plane (5) at A′. However, some (perhaps 25%) of the light from the edge B of the phosphor that is collected by the first lens misses the second lens so that the image at B′ is less bright. This is called vignetting, and occurs in the electron lens system also.

4.1.2 The television system

Camera tube

As Fig. 4.4(i) shows, the evacuated glass envelope of the camera tube, about 25 mm in diameter, contains:

- A signal plate (a), a thin transparent conductive layer, coated on the inside of the glass.

Over it is coated:

- A screen (b) containing a photoconducting mosaic (antimony trisulfide in the Vidicon tube and lead oxide in the Plumbicon tube). It converts the light pattern focused onto it into a pattern of electrical resistance.
- An electron gun (c), which sends a fine pencil of low-energy electrons, shown as a dashed line in the figure, toward the screen.

Time-varying voltages from a 'sweep generator' (SG) are applied to external coils (dd). They deflect the electron pencil so that it scans over the

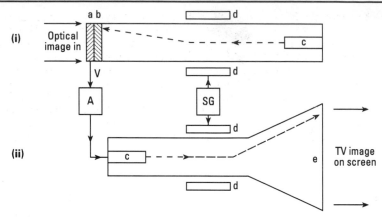

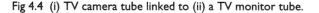

Fig 4.4 (i) TV camera tube linked to (ii) a TV monitor tube.

surface of the pick-up plate. As it passes over each element of the screen, a voltage ('video signal', V) is produced on the signal plate and varies according to the resistance at the point and so to the brightness of the incident image.

The signal does not respond instantly to a change of brightness. It shows a *lag*, which may be several hundred milliseconds. In comparison, the lag of the image intensifier tube is negligible, only 1 ms.

Monitor tube

The video signal V passes through an amplifier (A) to a TV monitor ('cathode ray') tube, shown in Fig. 4.4(ii). This evacuated glass envelope contains:

◆ at the narrow end, an electron gun (c), which projects a pencil of electrons, shown as a dashed line in the figure,
◆ a phosphor screen (e) coated on the inside of the wide end of the envelope, where the pencil produces a small dot of light.

The video signal from the camera tube is applied to the modulator or 'grid' of the electron gun and varies (modulates) the intensity of the electron stream and so the brightness of the spot of light on the monitor screen.

Time-varying voltages applied to external coils (dd) deflect the electron pencil so that it scans over the face of the phosphor in synchronism with the electron pencil in the camera tube. As it passes over each point, the brightness of the light produced varies directly as the brightness of the original image.

The electron pencil scans across the image in a raster of 625 horizontal lines, repeated 25 times a second. The scan is usually interlaced: alternate lines are 'written' in one 1/50 s and the other half in the next 1/50 s. The frame scan frequency is 50 Hz, in synchronism with the UK electric mains. The line frequency is $625 \times 25 \approx 15$ kHz, so that, typically, the spot moves with a 'writing speed' of 5–10 mm/µs. (The US standard is 525 lines at a frame scan frequency of 60 Hz.) The rectangular image has a height/width ratio of 4/3, which is ill-matched to the circular image produced by the image intensifier.

When moving from a high-attenuation to a low-attenuation area the increase in X-ray intensity could easily overload the TV system. This can be avoided in two ways. *Automatic gain control* uses the average video signal to control the average brightness of the video monitor and keep it constant. It can, however, deliver unnecessarily high doses to thinner parts and produce unnecessarily high noise in the image of thicker parts of the patient. Another limitation arises if it is used with an antiscatter grid and the grid is then removed. The gain will be automatically reduced to maintain the monitor brightness but the dose rate to the patient will remain the same. The other, preferred, method, automatic brightness control, is described in Section 4.1.3.

Video tape recording

The video signal is applied to the 'write' head of the recorder: a small coil which has a narrow gap in its closed iron core. This translates the video signal into a time-varying magnetic field. The signal is recorded as variations in the magnetism of the ferrous oxide coating of a plastic tape which travels at a high speed across the narrow gap. Switching from the 'write' or recording mode to the 'read' or playback mode, the traveling magnetic tape induces in the coil a voltage signal which, after amplication, reproduces the image on the TV monitor. Alternatively a video disk may be used.

Contrast and brightness can be varied as with any TV image. The dose to the patient is less than with cineradiography but the quality of the image is worse. No processing is needed; instant replay and frame freeze are possible.

4.1.3 Cameras

Cineradiography (e.g. of the heart)

A pulsed X-ray tube produces bursts of X-rays (pulse width 1–10 ms) only when the cine film is stationary. To avoid unproductive irradiation of the patient, no X-rays are produced while the film is being pulled through the camera gate between frames.

A pulsed (or grid-controlled) X-ray tube has the cathode hood insulated from the filament. Making the hood 2 kV negative cuts off the emission of electrons; while making it slightly positive effectively switches on the X-rays. A small (1 mm) focal spot and tube currents of 500–1000 mA are required, and the anode must have a high heat capacity.

Sixteen frames per second are sufficient to prevent jerky motion, but 50 frames/s are necessary to eliminate flicker. A high frame rate incurs a higher dose rate to expose each frame correctly. Each frame on a 35 mm film is 18 × 24 mm, and about a third of the circular field of the image is usually lost due to 'overframing'.

Automatic brightness control. The brightness of the image is monitored either by (a) measuring the (average) video signal or (b) by a sensor 'watching' the brightness of the output phosphor.

This ensures that the film is exposed within its latitude by controlling one or more of the following:

⬦ tube kilovoltage (kV);

⬦ tube milliamperage (mA), which is rather sluggish, but allows the operator free control of kV; or

⬦ pulse width, which allows free control of both kV and mA.

The same 'feedback' system is also used in fluoroscopy to control the brightness of the TV monitor automatically, as mentioned in the previous section. A dose–area monitor should also be used, for patient dose assurance.

Photospot film camera

This produces reduced size images, which are cheaper and easier to store, on 70 or 100 mm cut film, the partial mirror acting as a shutter in conjunction with pulsed X-rays. Five to 10 frames can be taken per second.

Due to the use of the image intensifier, the dose to the patient is, perhaps, 3–5 times smaller than with full-size (cassette-loaded) film, the exposure time shorter, and the movement blur less. The sharpness or resolution, being that of the image intensifier, is less good. One hundred millimeter film requires a greater patient dose than 70 mm.

4.1.4 Image quality

Resolution

Image quality in the brighter areas of the image is limited by blurring or poor spatial resolution. *Spatial resolution* is the ability to detect a single small structure against its background or to distinguish as separate two structures close together. It may be tested, as is done with broadcast TV, by imaging a bar 'test tool' or 'resolution grid'. As seen in Fig. 4.5a, this consists of a number of equally spaced bars, each space being the same as the width of a bar. In this case the bars are strips of lead affixed to a Perspex plate. A bar and a space together make up a line pair, and the spatial frequency of the pattern is the number of such *line pairs per millimeter* (lp mm^{-1}).

Figure 4.5a also plots the brightness of the screen image (or the video signal) along a scan line. (Plotting the density along a line across a film image produces a similar curve.) Blurring simply makes the edges unsharp, the contrast c being unaffected. Figure 4.5b illustrates a test grid of higher spatial frequency. The accompanying graph shows how the blurring now partially fills the gaps between the strips and reduces the contrast of the image to c'. The pattern is still visible, but it would not be if the blurring were greater. In Fig. 4.5c the test grid has an even higher spatial frequency. The blurrings merge in the gaps between the strips, the contrast is so much reduced, to C'', that the pattern 'disappears'.

Thus, if the blurring is too large or the bars too narrow and too close together, the blur of the edges of each bar merges with that of the adjacent one, and the gap between them cannot be distinguished.

Testing with patterns of several different frequencies, the spatial resolution of the system is defined as the spatial frequency of the finest pattern that can still be resolved.

The effect of blurring is to worsen resolution. The smaller the blurring the better the resolution. In film–screen radiography, for example, the film itself can resolve some 100 lp mm^{-1} whereas a slow ('detail') intensifying

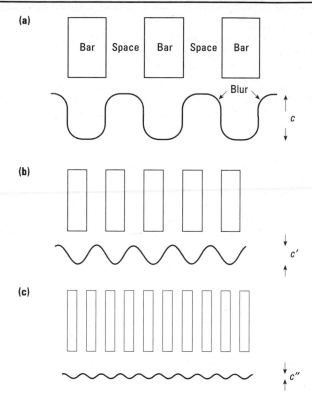

Fig. 4.5 Resolution test grids (a), (b) and (c) having different spatial frequencies and the corresponding plots of video signal or image brightness along a scan line, showing the effect of blurring on perceptibility.

screen can only resolve 10 lp mm^{-1}, and a fast screen 5 lp mm^{-1}. For further details see Section 9.3.

Resolution of the image intensifier. The image intensifier itself has a spatial resolution of about 4–5 lp mm^{-1} (or better in the magnification mode), and is principally affected by the blurring caused by light spread in the input phosphor (but not significantly in the much thinner output phosphor). Due to defects in the electron lens, the periphery of the image has worse resolution than the center. (It also shows greater magnification, which causes 'pincushion' distortion.)

The resolution is always stated in relation to the size of the X-ray image on the face of the intensifier. The resolution with 100 mm cut film is nearly as good but, on 35 mm film is only about half as good, as that of the intensifier itself.

Resolution of the TV system. The TV system degrades the resolution further due to the mosaic structure of the TV camera image plate and to two aspects of the way in which the image is scanned:

◈ *Line structure.* The line structure of the TV image affects vertical resolution. The latter is tested with the test pattern positioned with the bars horizontal. Since the image is composed of 625 horizontal lines, one might expect to be able to resolve a total of 625 alternate 'black' and 'white' lines (312 line pairs).

In fact (partly because in practice not all the 625 lines are used to form the image but mainly because of the way the eye performs) only about 200 line pairs can be resolved in the vertical direction. When these are spread over a 230 mm field, the vertical resolution is about 1 lp mm^{-1}. With the smaller fields, in magnification mode, the resolution is better.

There would be no point in photographing the monitor screen on account of the poor resolution compared with photographing the output phosphor.

◆ *Bandwidth*. The bandwidth of the TV monitor electronics affects horizontal resolution.

The bandwidth is the maximum frequency of alternation of the video signal that can be handled without distortion. To match the above resolution when the test pattern is turned with the bars vertical, the system has to cope with 260 alternations between black and white along each scan line, when account is taken of the rectangular shape of the screen. It has to do so 625×25 times a second, a total of 4 million alternations per second or 4 MHz. The TV system normally used would have a bandwidth of up to 10 MHz, which is about twice that of broadcast TV.

Interlacing is not entirely satisfactory; resolution may be impaired if tissues move between the two halves of a 1/25 s frame. A high-resolution image intensifier (II)–TV system employs 1250 lines, noninterlaced ('progressive') scan, can resolve 2 lp mm^{-1}, produces a square image, but requires a bandwidth of at least 25 MHz. Digital photospot imaging (see Section 4.2.1) produces high resolution with the normal bandwidth.

Contrast

In the image intensifier, contrast may be impaired by backward-traveling light, which penetrates the aluminum film and excites the photocathode. It may also be reduced by X-rays penetrating the input screen and falling on the output phosphor.

Veiling glare is due to scattering of light, particularly in the output window of the image intensifier, and to a lesser extent in the TV camera tube. (It is similar to the scattering and reflection of light within the body of a camera lens, known as 'flare'.) It reduces the contrast of the image in much the same way as scattered X-rays in radiography. It is worse with the larger sizes of intensifier.

An image intensifier can be tested by imaging a lead disk which covers the central 10% of its front face. Its shadow (which should be totally dark) is commonly 1/20 or 1/30 as bright as the surrounding field.

A Vidicon camera has $\gamma = 0.8$ while a Plumbicon tube has $\gamma = 1.0$. The γ-value of the TV monitor system can be varied, up to 2.0, so that the contrast is, on the whole, increased.

Dynamic range (latitude) of the television monitor

This is the ratio

$$\frac{\text{maximum acceptable brightness of the TV monitor screen}}{\text{smallest detectable brightness above black}}$$

and is typically 1000:1, which is usually expressed as 30 dB, as explained

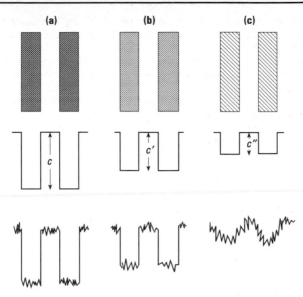

Fig. 4.6 Resolution tests grids (a), (b) and (c) having different inherent contrasts and the corresponding plots of video signal or image brightness along a scan line, showing the effect of noise on perceptibility.

in Section 7.16. The choice of kV and the setting of the TV contrast control are made so that the range of tissues being imaged fall within the dynamic range.

Noise

Quantum mottle is noticeable in fluoroscopy, unlike radiography. Image quality in the less bright areas of the image is limited by noise – the statistical fluctuations in the number of X-ray photons absorbed in the input phosphor. This in turn produces similar fluctuations in the brightness of the image, the density recorded on a spot film and the video signal voltage from the camera tube. Noise reduces the perceptibility of a structure having low contrast.

Figure 4.6 depicts part of each of three resolution grids having (a) high, (b) medium, and (c) low contrast, made perhaps with strips of lead, aluminum, and Perpsex, respectively. To simplify matters we assume that any blurring is negligible. Below each test grid is the corresponding image brightness or video signal plotted along a scan line, in the absence of noise. In each case, c indicates the contrast.

Beneath that we see the same signal with superimposed noise, which effectively reduces the contrast. The bars can easily be resolved in Fig. 4.6a. They can still be resolved in Fig. 4.6b, *but they would not be if the noise were greater*. In Fig. 4.6c the contrast is completely obscured and the bars cannot be distinguished from the spaces between them. Thus, if the noise is too great, the contrast difference is too small, or the structures are too small, or too close together, the structures cannot be distinguished.

With a typical average dose rate in air of 1–2 μGy s^{-1} on the surface of the image intensifier, during the 1/6 s time constant (lag) of a Vidicon camera tube, an average of 3000 X-ray photons might be absorbed in each square millimeter of the input phosphor. As a result, when trying to see a structure 1 mm^2 in size, the noise is √3000, which is 2% of the signal. The signal-to-noise ratio (SNR) is 50:1. Now it turns out that, for a structure to be detectable, the contrast must at least be some 2–5 times the noise relative to signal. So a structure 1 mm in size will be seen against its background provided its contrast is at least 5%.

The image of a small structure is produced by the absorption of relatively few photons and is noisy, and to see it requires a high contrast. Either a high dose rate is used to increase the SNR, or the inherent contrast of the object has to be increased, e.g by changing the kV or using a contrast medium.

The image of a broader structure is produced by the absorption of more photons and has less noise, and to see it does not require so high a contrast. Objects larger than 1 mm are detectable even when their contrasts are less than 5%. Their visibility is ultimately noise limited.

The foregoing is illustrated by Fig. 4.7, in which the solid curve plots on a logarithmic scale the minimum contrast needed to see, i.e. resolve, structures of different diameters. It is obtained by using a specially constructed test object (e.g. Leeds TO 10) with an image intensifier. Details having a size and contrast falling in region A can be resolved; those falling in region B cannot. The dashed line shows the improvement in perceptibility produced by increasing the dose rate and so reducing noise.

To summarize:

◆ the contrast resolution (the smallest detectable contrast) improves with larger details;
◆ the spatial resolution improves with higher contrast;
◆ increasing the dose rate reduces noise and improves the inherent detectability of all structures.

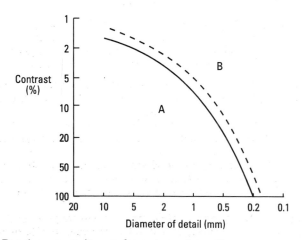

Fig. 4.7 Detail–contrast diagram for an image intensifier.

This relationship (or 'trade-off') between spatial resolution, contrast and noise or dose applies to all forms of imaging (digital, computed tomography (CT) gamma, etc.). In film–screen radiography, however, noise is usually too small to affect the perception of detail.

The lag in a Vidicon camera tube smooths out the statistical fluctuations and reduces noise or mottle. A Plumbicon tube shows less lag and less movement blurring but more noise than a Vidicon tube.

The noise is worse in the areas of the image where the brightness is low. It could be improved by increasing the tube current and X-ray intensity, but this would unduly increase patient dose. The quality of the image is said to be *dose limited* or *photon limited*.

On the other hand, full advantage cannot be taken of the brightness gain of an image intensifier in the reduction of patient dose. The mA cannot be reduced much below that formerly used in direct vision fluoroscopy, as to do so would increase noise unduly. Even so, due to the brighter image the contrast and definition present in the image *can actually be seen*, in higher ambient lighting and by more than one viewer. This is the real advantage of the image intensifier.

Typical doses and dose rates

Images with acceptable noise are produced by the following approximate doses and dose rates on the input surface of the image intensifier:

Fluoroscopy	$1 \ \mu Gy \ s^{-1}$
Photospot film	$1 \ \mu Gy \ frame^{-1}$
Cine	$0.1 \ \mu Gy \ frame^{-1}$
Digital	$10 \ \mu Gy \ frame^{-1}$

Due to attenuation by the patient, grid, and couch top, the skin proximal to the tube will receive doses around $300 \times$ greater. See also Section 6.7.

Quantum sink

The information in the image also suffers from statistical fluctuations in all the other discrete 'events' occurring in the image chain:

> light photons emitted by the input phosphor
> → photoelectrons emitted by the photocathode
> → light photons emitted by the output phosphor
> → electrons constituting the video signal, etc.

The noise produced in each of the above stages is relatively low since, due to the intensification process described in Section 4.1.1, the number of light photons and electrons involved is very large.

That part of the system where the number of photons or electrons per square millimeter of the image field is least, the relative noise therefore the largest and the SNR the lowest, is known as the quantum sink. It is the weakest link in the imaging chain, and nothing that happens closer to the viewer than the quantum sink can increase the amount of real information in the image; although it can makes its appearance better.

In an II–TV system, the quantum sink lies in the absorption of X-rays in the input phosphor. In radiography, it lies in the absorption of X-rays in the intensifying screens.

4.2 DIGITAL IMAGING

The radiological images considered so far are analog images. In particular, the video signal from the TV camera tube is an analog signal, a voltage which varies smoothly as the image brightness is scanned in the raster of horizontal lines. If it is converted to digital form, the image can be enhanced in various ways – and if necessary stored – using a computer, before it is displayed on a video monitor or printed via a laser camera.

4.2.1 Equipment

Digitizer

The video signal from the TV camera is applied to an analog–digital converter (ADC) or digitizer. This samples the signal at equally spaced intervals (say) 512 times along each of 512 scan lines. Figure 4.8 shows how the video signal varies during the time it takes to scan a single line and how it is sampled at regular intervals. The voltage at each data point, which gives the grey level, is expressed as the nearest 10-bit binary number between,

00000 00000 (=0) and 11111 11111 (= 1023)

(An explanation of binary numbers is given in Section 4.5.)

Computer

The image has in effect been divided into a matrix of 512 × 512 pixels, depicted in Fig. 4.9a. Each pixel is roughly a square of side 0.5 mm. This permits a resolution of 1 mm (= two pixels). The same diagram can be taken to represent a corresponding 'frame' of 512 × 512 memory locations in the core memory of a computer (microprocessor).

The binary numbers representing the image brightness or 'grey level' of each pixel are stored in a frame of 512 × 512 memory locations. Each location has an 'address', expressed as two binary numbers and is '10 bits deep'. This requires a storage capacity of 10 × 512 × 512 bits = 320 kilobytes (where 1 byte = 8 bits). Thus a 40 megabyte RAM (random access memory) can store 128 separate images.

If the sampling frequency were to be doubled, to 1024 per scan line, the pixel size would be halved, the matrix size doubled, and the resolution

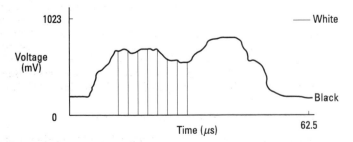

Fig. 4.8 Sampling and digitization of a video signal along a scan line.

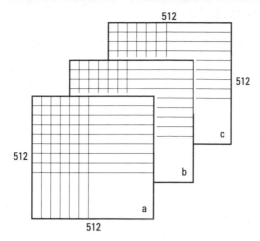

Fig. 4.9 Three successive image frames of a digital image, each a matrix of pixels or memory locations.

improved by a factor of 2. However, the 40 megabyte RAM could then only store 30 separate images. For further remarks about sampling frequency, see Section 9.2.

Image display

The image is displayed by reading out of the computer memory the brightness or grey scale values of the pixels in sequence, in synchronism with the electron pencil scanning the monitor (cathode ray tube). The data from the computer are converted (by a digital–analog convertor, DAC) into an analog voltage signal which modulates the brightness of the spot of light on the screen.

Last frame hold. A simple application is to store ('freeze frame') the last image of a fluoroscopic examination so that it can continue to be observed on the monitor without continuing to expose the patient.

Digital photospot: high-resolution, slow television scan

A very short exposure at high mA is made, thus freezing movement. The video system is made inoperative ('blanked') during the actual exposure. The camera then scans the image and writes it into the computer memory with a 1024 line progressive (noninterlaced) raster at 6.25 frames s^{-1} – four times more slowly than normal – thus allowing the usual bandwidth to be used. The stored image is read out of the memory at the usual 25 frames s^{-1} for flicker-free display on a monitor or is recorded with a laser camera, described below. The spatial resolution is typically 2 lp mm^{-1}, compared with 4 lp mm^{-1} for an ordinary photospot, but with the advantages of digital imaging.

4.2.2 Image processing, storage, and recording

Before reading out the stored image from memory, the grey scale numbers in each address can be processed and manipulated in a number of ways.

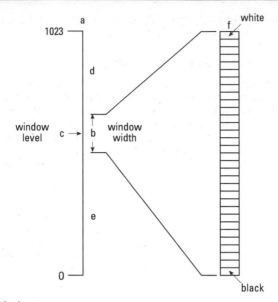

Fig. 4.10 Windowing.

Windowing

The digitized image contains more information than can be seen at once on the monitor screen. The image stored in a 10-bit computer contains 1024 discrete intensity levels, represented by scale a in Fig. 4.10, but the eye can only distinguish about 32 gradations of brightness on a TV screen.

A small range of values b, the window width, centered on the window level c, is selected for display on the monitor as (say) 32 distinct shades of grey f in the range from black to maximum white. Intensities in the range d are not differentiated, being all displayed as white, while those in the range e are all displayed as black.

It is possible to visualize subject contrast only in the structures or tissues whose image lies within the *window width*. The *window level* is the mid-range value of the window, and it and the window width can be independently set at the controls. By moving the window level into the image areas d or e, these parts of the image then become differentiated and can be visualized.

Windowing is sometimes called 'grey level mapping'. It allows the contrast and the average brightness of the image to be optimized within the tissues and region of interest. In effect it allows the speed and γ or latitude of the imaging system to be altered at will, subsequent to a single X-ray exposure – something which cannot be done in film–screen radiography. This feature can outweigh the poorer resolution of digital compared with film–screen radiography.

Background subtraction

Subtraction of the same number from each of the stored pixel values will increase contrast. (This is the opposite of the effect of scatter or fog reducing contrast on a radiograph.) This technique can be used to reduce the effect of X-ray scattering and veiling glare.

Noise reduction by frame addition or averaging

Several successive images of the same subject, stored in memory, are added together and averaged, pixel by pixel. The useful signals are in the same locations in all frames and so will add up. The noise varies randomly from frame to frame and is therefore partially averaged out. As a result, the SNR is improved by a factor equal to the square root of the number of frames so averaged. This is sometimes called 'digital temporal filtering'. It depends on the patient being immobile while the several images are acquired.

Noise reduction by 'low-pass spatial filtering'

To the grey scale value of each pixel is added a proportion of the pixel values of the eight surrounding pixels and an average taken. This reduces noise but can impair spatial resolution. Small bright or dark areas are removed whether they are noise or real images, while leaving the images of larger objects. It can be compared to turning up the bass control of a hi-fi system. Digital filtering is further explained in Section 9.1.

Edge enhancement by 'high-pass spatial filtering'

Where the pixel values change at an edge or boundary in the image, the gradient can be enhanced mathematically. (It achieves digitally the edge enhancement feature inherent in xerography – described in Section 3.11.) It can be used to reduce the effect of blurring in the imaging system. It will therefore enhance those parts of the image with fine structure detail, but in doing so it increases noise. It can be compared with turning up the treble control of a hi-fi system.

Data shifting

The pixel values can be moved horizontally and/or vertically within a frame, and the image can be shifted, inverted, rotated, or even stretched.

Image storage

A number of separate images can be stored in real time, usually in a solid state memory (RAM). Access to stored images is rapid (microseconds) but the storage capacity is limited by cost. To make the RAM available for further images, the stored data are transferred to a magnetic disk. This is a medium-term store and may be either a floppy disk, which is portable but has a storage capacity of only about 1 megabyte, or a hard (Winchester) disk able to store several thousand images. Access is reasonably fast (milliseconds).

For long-term storage (archiving) the images are transferred to optical disks which have a capacity of many gigabytes. The digital information is burnt by a laser into a specially coated disk. They are the cheapest form of storage. Digital magnetic tape storage is also used, and has a very high storage capacity (optical tape is even better), but again access is relatively slow.

When required, digitally stored images can be played back into the solid state memory and, after any necessary manipulation, displayed on the screen. A series of still images can be presented in rapid sequence ('cine' mode).

Cameras

The image on the monitor screen can be recorded on single-coated photographic film which has been formulated so that its spectral sensitivity matches the light emitted by the cathode ray tube phosphor, and it can be processed in the normal X-ray film automatic processor.

To obtain good images the cathode ray tube must be of a high grade and the film correctly exposed. This is achieved by a light sensor attached to a corner of the screen which feeds back to the modulator grid of the electron gun and controls the brightness of the screen.

A *laser camera* can be connected directly to the digital processor, bypassing the cathode ray tube. A helium–neon gas laser (for example) emits a beam of light only (say) 70 µm in diameter. This is scanned in a raster across a moving film by means of a rotating or oscillating mirror and so records the image. The image is recorded by reading out of the memory the brightness or grey scale values of the pixels in sequence, in synchronism with the laser beam scanning the recording film. The data from the computer are converted (by a DAC) into an analog voltage signal which modulates the brightness of the laser beam. It takes a total of 20 s to scan a film, which, on account of the narrow laser beam, can record about 4096×4096 pixels, with a resolution of 10 lp mm^{-1}. The single-coated film is specially formulated for infrared and the automatic processor. A green safelight may be used.

In a *multiformat camera* (whether conventional or laser) the whole of the screen image can be made to fill either the whole film or just a part of it, in which latter case a number of images may be recorded, reduced in size, side by side.

The above methods of processing, storing, and recording a digital image all find general application in CT, gamma imaging, digital ultrasound, and magnetic resonance imaging.

4.2.3 Digital subtraction angiography

The object of digital subtraction angiography is to produce images of contrast-filled vessels in isolation from other tissues and with the minimum of contrast medium. Images of the same region are taken in rapid succession, before and after injection of a contrast medium, while avoiding any movement of the patient or equipment. The video signals are converted electronically to their logarithms (to match the exponential attenuation of X-rays in tissue) and then digitized. Then, as illustrated schematically in Fig. 4.11:

(1) The mask or non-contrast image (a) is taken before the contrast medium has reached the target area. It shows normal anatomy only, and is stored as one frame in the computer memory.
(2) The contrast (or enhanced) image (b) is taken when the vessels have filled with contrast medium. It shows filled vessels superimposed on normal anatomy and is stored as a second frame.

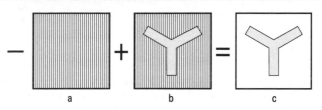

Fig. 4.11 Subtraction angiography (schematic). (a) Non-contrast, (b) contrast and (c) subtraction images.

(3) The two images are 'registered', by data shifting, and then subtracted, pixel by pixel. The resulting subtraction image (c) is stored as a third frame. This shows the filled vessels only.

After windowing and digital-to-analog conversion, the subtraction image is displayed on the monitor. As a result of this process, the parts of the contrast image which coincide with the mask image (bones and soft tissues) have been eliminated from the subtraction image, leaving only the vessels filled with contrast medium.

Conversion of the video signal to its logarithm matches the exponential absorption of the primary beam, but it is not so appropriate for scattered radiation. The computer program can partly compensate for the effect of scatter (and similarly that of veiling glare) on the subtraction image.

Digital subtraction angiography generally requires:

◆ a large field (300 mm) image intensifier with good contrast resolution;
◆ a very stable TV system with low noise and small lag;
◆ an X-ray tube with a reasonably small focal spot; and
◆ a high-voltage generator with an exceptionally stable output, capable of giving a large number of very short (30–100 ms) exposures in rapid sequence (2–8 frames s^{-1}).

To reduce quantum noise to an acceptable level, the mA is switched to a value some 100 times greater than the usual screening current. Simultaneously, an iris diaphragm between the lenses must be stopped down, so as not to overload the TV camera. This, together with pulsing the X-ray tube and energizing the motor-driven syringe, are all under the control of the same computer which stores and processes the data.

Noise

The quantum noise in the subtraction image is greater than the noise in either the mask or contrast images. The signals subtract but the noises reinforce, thereby reducing the SNR. The noise in the mask image can be reduced by obtaining and storing a sequence of such images and then summing them pixel by pixel. The images add together but the random noise tends to average out. The relative noise is reduced, and the SNR is increased by a factor equal to the square root of the number of images that are averaged. The noise in the contrast image can be reduced similarly.

Temporal subtraction

This is the process so far described. Images can be spoiled by movement of tissues due to breathing, swallowing, peristalsis, cardiac motion, vascular pulsations, etc. Motion artefacts can often be eliminated by realigning the images with pixel shifting before subtracting them. Another method of eliminating these artefacts uses energy subtraction, which avoids the need for a mask image.

Energy subtraction

Suppose it were possible to take two images of the iodine-filled vessels with monoenergetic X-rays of 32 and 34 keV, respectively, either side of the K-edge of iodine. The attenuation and contrast of iodine would differ markedly between the two images while those of bone and soft tissue would hardly change. Subtracting the images would eliminate both bone and soft tissue, leaving only the iodine image.

In practice, using heterogeneous beams it is possible to eliminate only one of the tissues. An exposure is made at a high kV (say 140 kV) and the image is stored. Very rapidly, to avoid motion artefacts, the generator is switched to a lower kV (say 65 kV) and a higher mA, and a second exposure is made and the image stored. The two images have different bone–soft tissue contrast and can be subtracted in different proportions in such a way as to eliminate either bone or soft tissue. An alternative method of energy subtraction uses two different K-edge filters to shape the spectra.

Hybrid subtraction

Two mask images are taken in rapid succession at different kV values and then energy subtracted to eliminate soft tissue, leaving bone. After an appropriate interval, two contrast images are taken in rapid succession at different kV values and energy subtracted to eliminate soft tissue, leaving bone and contrast medium. The two resulting images are then subtracted (temporally), eliminating bone and leaving the vessel filled with contrast medium. In this technique, artefacts due to movement of soft tissues are eliminated. The three subtractions have, however, increased the noise in the image.

4.2.4 Quality assurance

In addition to the tube and generator tests described in Section 2.7.5 and the image quality tests applicable to fluoroscopy (see Section 4.1.4), specially designed test objects should be used to check the greater sensitivity and masking – or subtraction – capabilities of digital subtraction angiography.

4.3 COMPUTED TOMOGRAPHY (CT)

In CT scanning:

(a) A transverse slice of the patient, for example 10 mm thick, shown schematically in Fig. 4.12. is imaged, thus avoiding the superposition of adjacent structures that occurs in conventional radiography.

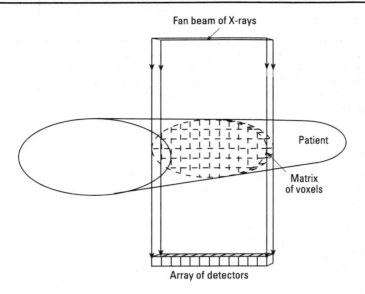

Fan beam of X-rays

Patient

Matrix
of voxels

Array of detectors

Fig. 4.12 Principle of CT imaging.

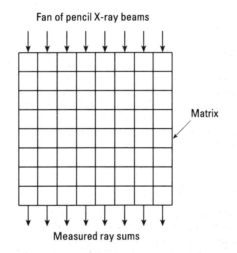

Fan of pencil X-ray beams

Matrix

Measured ray sums

Fig. 4.13 Matrix of tissue voxels, corresponding memory locations in the computer or pixels in the image.

(b) The slice is defined by a 'sheet' of X-rays, produced by a narrow fan beam rotated around the patient, thus reducing the amount of scatter produced.

(c) The slice is in effect subdivided as shown, into a matrix of 512 × 512 volume elements (voxels), each typically 0.5 × 0.5 × 10 mm. The image is reconstructed by a digital computer as a corresponding matrix of 512 × 512 picture elements (pixels) represented in Fig. 4.13.

(d) The computer allows the use of 'windowing' (see Section 4.2.2) to selectively display a restricted range of tissues.

On account of (a), (b), and (d) the contrast resolution, the ability to display low contrast structures, is better than in conventional radiography; but on account of (c) the spatial resolution is less good.

The image is displayed as a matrix of pixels, each 0.5×0.5 mm. Note that the pixel size is not the size on the screen, but is the size referred to the X-ray field or body being imaged. The brightness or grey scale value of each pixel in the image represents the average linear attenuation coefficient μ of the contents of the corresponding voxel.

4.3.1 Principle of computed tomography imaging

CT numbers

The linear attenuation coefficient μ_t of each tissue pixel is compared with that μ_w of water by the formula:

$$\text{CT number} = 1000(\mu_t - \mu_w)/\mu_w$$

Water is used as the reference material because its attenuation coefficient is close to those of soft tissues and it is a reproducible material for machine calibration. The multiplier (1000) is used to obtain whole numbers.

The CT number (or Hounsfield number) is defined as −1000 for air and 0 for water; for tissues it depends on the kV employed. For example if, at 80 keV, the linear attenuation coefficients of typical bone and water are 0.38 and 0.19 cm^{-1}, respectively, the CT number of the bone is +1000. It can be higher in the case of cortical bone. Other representative values are indicated in Fig. 4.16 but they vary from machine to machine.

Scanning the patient

In the commonest form of CT scanner, sketched in Fig. 4.17c, a rotating anode tube with a 0.6 mm focal spot is employed. It must have a high heat capacity because only a slice of the X-ray beam is used and the examination time may take several seconds. The tube is mounted with its axis perpendicular to the slice, to reduce any heel effect.

The X-rays are collimated as they leave the tube into a fan beam which just covers the body section. After emerging from the patient the transmitted beam passes through a second collimator set, accurately aligned with the first; both sets being motorized to set the slice thickness. The beam then falls on a curvilinear array of (say) 700 detectors, individually collimated and all carefully matched as to sensitivity. These convert the transmitted beam intensity into a proportional signal current.

The tube and detectors, mounted on opposite sides of a ring, rotate smoothly around the patient. In the course of a 360° rotation, the X-ray tube is pulsed some 300 times. Each pulse of X-rays lasts 2–3 ms, and the scan can take about 1 s.

Figures 4.12 and 4.13 represent the matrix of tissue voxels traversed by the fan beam of X-rays which are then incident on the array of detectors. For simplicity, the detectors, at the bottom of Fig. 4.12 have been drawn as a linear array, and in Fig. 4.13 the pencil beams of the fan have been drawn parallel. The computer is able to allow for the fact that they diverge and that the diverging fan does not 'match' the square array of pixels.

Acquiring the data

Each time the tube is pulsed, each detector, and its associated electronics, measures the logarithm of the intensity of the radiation falling upon it. These figures are related to the sum of all the CT numbers of the voxels each ray has passed through, which is called the ray sum. (The set of ray sums collected at each position of the tube is called a projection.) The large number of ray sums are temporarily stored in the computer. The computer allows for the fact that, if a pencil beam of width t passes obliquely through a pixel of size $t \times t$, some of the contents of the pixel will be 'missed'.

Figure 4.13 represents only one position of the fan beam. Each individual voxel is in fact traversed by an X-ray pencil from several different directions during the 360° rotation of the ring. The CT number of each voxel then features in several of the ray sums measured.

Reconstructing the image

In principle, if we have 256×256 voxels and 700×300 ray sums we have more than enough simultaneous equations to solve for the individual CT numbers of all of the voxels. The arithmetic involved can be performed in a sufficiently short time only by a computer and by taking various short cuts, one of which ('filtered back-projection') is described below. In this way the CT image can be produced in close to real time.

The CT numbers so computed are stored in the computer memory locations, each of which corresponds to a voxel and therefore to a pixel, as in Fig. 4.13.

Back-projection

Consider for simplicity one voxel, the contents of which have a higher μ than its surroundings. As depicted in Fig. 4.14a, an X-ray pencil traverses the voxel and the ray sum is measured. In principle, a stripe of light could now be projected backward along the direction of the X-ray, skimming the surface of the page, its intensity being proportional to the ray sum.

Repeating this for each of the rays which traverse the voxel in the course of a scan would build up an image of the structure (Fig. 4.14b). With a moderate number of stripes the image would be rather spiky (Fig. 4.14c). As the number of stripes increases, the spikiness would develop into a blurring of the edges of the image (Fig. 4.14d). The blurring could be removed by modifying the brightness near the edges of each back-projected beam or stripe – a process known as 'filtering'.

The foregoing is simply an analogy. In fact, the above procedure is carried out in purely arithmetical terms by the computer. A highly simplified version is given in Fig. 4.15, in which an array of nine pixels is scanned from four successive directions (Fig. 4.15a–d), in each case producing the ray sums shown. The three ray sums in Fig. 4.15a are entered (as in Fig. 4.14e) into the memory locations corresponding to each of the voxels encountered by each ray. Similarly the rays sums shown in Fig. 4.15b–d are back-projected in Fig. 4.15f–h, respectively. Adding the numbers (Fig. 4.15e–h), so entered in each memory location results in the totals shown in Fig. 4.15i. A little further arithmetic manipulation, involving background subtraction and rescaling, finally yields Fig. 4.15k. This is a fair representation of the CT numbers of each pixel (compare with the ray sums of Fig. 4.15a–d).

Filtered back-projection. The blurring introduced by the back-projection

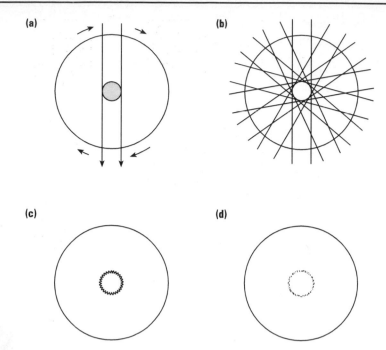

Fig. 4.14 Back-projection: schematic. (a) Pencil beam rotating around a small dense structure. (b)-(d) Image reconstructed with increasing numbers of projections.

process can be compensated by a mathematical process, carried out by the computer, called 'filtering'. This effectively modifies the brightness near the edge of each back-projected beam, as explained in Section 5.8.1. Different 'filters' can be used, formulated to make it easier either to detect low-contrast objects or to enhance resolution in bone. (See also Section 4.3.3.)

Windowing

Although the scanner can distinguish 2000 different CT numbers, as shown in the left-hand scale in Fig. 4.16, the eye cannot distinguish nearly as many separate shades of grey on the screen. In any case, as the figure shows, soft tissues (excluding fat) only cover a range of about 80 CT numbers.

So a window is chosen, as described in Section 4.2.2, which just embraces all the tissues of interest, and only these are displayed as shades of grey within the range black to maximum white available on the monitor. As depicted in Fig. 4.16, pixels with CT numbers outside this window are undifferentiated, being displayed as either black or white. Window level and window width can be set independently at the control panel, for example to differentiate lung tissues or bone. The window settings are displayed digitally on the screen. They only affect the displayed image; the whole of the data referring to the reconstructed image is retained in the computer.

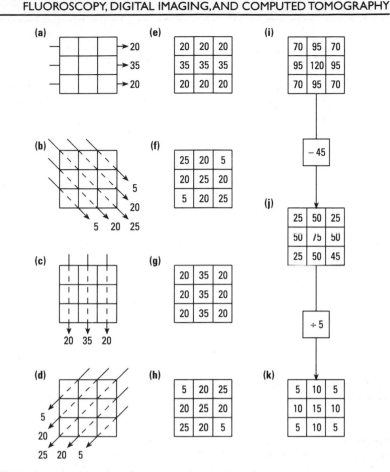

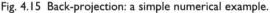
Fig. 4.15 Back-projection: a simple numerical example.

Partial volume effect

CT cannot reveal detail within a voxel. It measures the average CT number of the contents of each voxel. A high-contrast object occupying only part of a voxel will raise the CT number for the corresponding pixel and so appear larger than it is. Tiny calcifications and small traces of contrast medium are made visible in this way. The partial volume effect may be reduced by using a thinner slice and smaller pixels.

Beam-hardening effect

The use of a relatively high kV (typically 120 kV constant potential) reduces both patient dose and the hardening of the beam by the patient. Unfortunately, it reduces the efficiency of the detector and also the contrast of the image. It also increases scatter, making necessary the collimation in front of the detectors.

Hardening of the beam as it penetrates the patient results in the CT number of the same kind of tissue decreasing along the ray. However, the

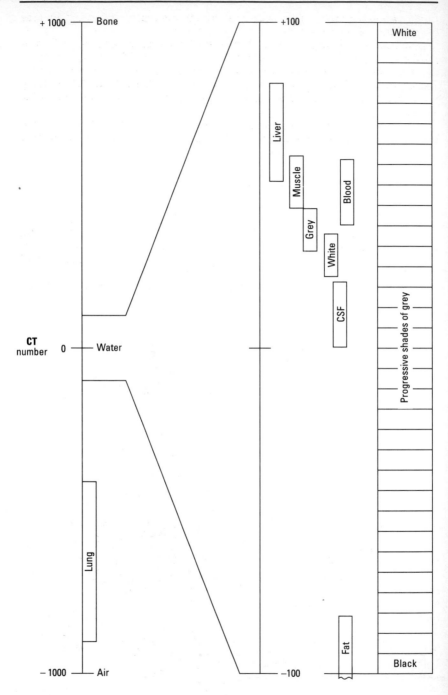

Fig. 4.16 Windowing in CT.

image reconstruction process assumes that, to the contrary, the CT number of each kind of tissue is constant along each ray.

This beam-hardening effect is allowed for by the computer using a 'beam-hardening algorithm', and is reduced by the use of a 0.5 mm copper filter mounted on the X-ray tube, which, with the high kV, produces a relatively homogeneous beam. Recently, improved beam-hardening algorithms have allowed lighter filtration, resulting in a greater tube output and a shorter scan time.

To compensate for the diminishing patient thickness toward the edges of the fan beam, a 'bow tie' compensating filter, thicker along two parallel edges than in the center, may be used.

4.3.2 The computed tomography scanner

Configurations

The *first-generation scanner* (Fig. 4.17a) used a single pencil beam falling on a single detector; together they translated through 180 steps and then rotated 1° at a time through 360°, taking a total scan time for one slice of 3–5 min.

The *second-generation scanner* (Fig. 4.17b) used a narrow fan beam

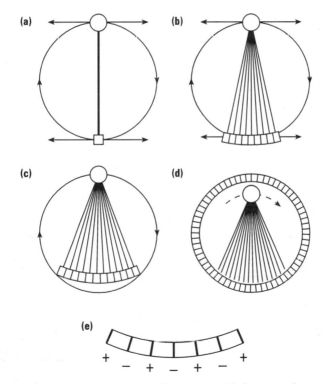

Fig. 4.17 (a)–(d) Four generations of CT scanner. (e) Portion of a curvilinear gas ionization detector array.

falling on a small curved array of detectors; together they translated and then rotated through 360° but needed fewer angular steps to produce the image, thus reducing the scan time to 20 s per slice.

The *third-generation scanner* (Fig. 4.17c), the one most frequently used, and described earlier, employs a wide fan beam falling on a larger array of many hundreds of detectors which do not translate but simply rotate continuously through 360° around the patient. The scan time is reduced to 1 s. The tube and detectors are always in the same geometrical relation, allowing better predetector collimation but making the image subject to ring artefacts.

In the *fourth-generation scanner* (Fig. 4.17d), the X-ray tube alone rotates through 360° around the patient, who is positioned within a continuous ring of several thousands of stationary detectors. It is no faster, but ring artefacts are avoided. It is easier to calibrate (i.e. monitor the sensitivity of) the detectors continually using the leading and trailing edge of the fan beam. The tube is closer to the patient than the detectors, which is the reverse of the ideal, and radiation doses to the patient are higher.

Slip-ring technology. If the tube kV is supplied by high-tension cables, the gantry ring has to reverse direction after each 360° rotation. Faster continuous rotation of the tube is achieved in modern scanners by mounting a high-voltage generator, operating at high frequency (up to 100 kHz) and therefore light and compact, on the rotating gantry ring itself and supplying it with power though slip-rings. The tube can rotate in one direction indefinitely, thus making possible *helical scanning* (see Section 4.3.4).

Further increase of scan speed is possible by simultaneous use of multiple X-ray tubes or by inserting the patient into a huge funnel-shaped X-ray tube in which an electron beam (1000 mA) scans rapidly round a large semicircular target – usually called the *fifth-generation scanner*. Multiple stationary detector rings allow multiple slices to be scanned simultaneously. A scan time of 50–100 ms eliminates motion artefacts in cardiac imaging or when voluntary breath holding is not possible.

Detectors

The detectors need to have:

- high-detection efficiency;
- fast response (short afterglow) to keep up with fast scanning;
- wide dynamic range – able to cope with both the high-intensity beam either side of the patient and the highly attenuated beam passing through the patient (intensity ratio 5000:1);
- linearity – signal accurately proportional to the X-ray intensity;
- stability in face of voltage and temperature fluctuations;
- reliability;
- small size to allow close packing, giving better resolution;
- low cost in view of the large number of detectors used.

Scintillators. Originally a sodium iodide (thallium-activated) crystal was used, coupled to a photomultiplier which required a highly stabilized high-voltage power supply. (The principle is the same as used in a gamma camera, described in Section 5.3.) Sodium iodide has been superseded by other scintillators with shorter afterglow such as cesium iodide, calcium fluoride, cadmium tungstate, and bismuth germanate. Photomultipliers have been superseded by very much smaller silicon photodiodes, which do not need a high-voltage supply. Very close packing can be achieved with crystals of cadmium tungstate or cesium iodide, with a silicon light sensor embedded in each solid state detector.

Ionization chambers. Ionization chambers are less sensitive but more easily matched for sensitivity. They are very stable, unaffected by voltage fluctuations, and have a wide linear response with no lag. They are narrow (and closely packed) but are made relatively deep, to increase sensitivity. For which reason also they are filled with a high atomic number gas (xenon) at high pressure (25 atm, 2.5 MPa) rather than air. The tungsten electrodes, alternately positive and negative (Fig. 4.17e), converge toward the tube (like the strips in a focused grid), and so help to collimate the beam and reduce scatter.

Ionization chambers are therefore well suited to third-generation scanners, where very stable detectors are needed as their sensitivity cannot be checked or calibrated very often. They are less suitable for fourth-generation scanners as the electrode plates would have to converge to the center of the ring. Solid state detectors are more appropriate, particularly as their sensitivity can be checked continuously by the leading or trailing edge of the X-ray fan beam.

4.3.3 Image quality

Noise

Even when the scanner is operating properly, the image is not uniform but appears mottled or grainy. This can be tested by imaging a water phantom. The CT numbers of the pixels will not be all the same, due to statistical variations in the number of X-ray photons absorbed in each voxel. The computer can be asked to compute the mean CT number and also the standard deviation or noise.

The quantum noise is a fundamental limit to the quality of the CT image since it both reduces contrast resolution of small objects and worsens the spatial resolution of low-contrast objects.

Noise may be reduced by increasing the number of photons absorbed in each voxel, by increasing the slice thickness or the pixel size. However, improving contrast resolution in this way will impair spatial resolution. Noise can also be reduced by increasing either the mA or the scan time. However, both of these involve increasing the patient dose. To minimize patient dose the radiologist must accept the noisiest picture consistent with good diagnosis.

Other factors affecting noise. Zoom enlargement of the display spreads the available ray sum information more thinly over the pixel matrix and therefore increases noise. Using a narrower window also makes noise more noticeable, as each grey level covers a smaller range of CT numbers, i.e. is derived from the absorption of fewer X-ray photons in each voxel.

Reducing the scan time or reducing the slice thickness also involves an increase in noise, unless the mA is increased proportionally. There is a deficiency of photons, and noise is accordingly worse with thicker patients and also when there are high-attenuation materials such as bone or prostheses in the slice.

Spatial resolution of high-contrast objects

High-contrast spatial resolution is good, being determined by pixel size. In CT terms 'high contrast' is that between water and Perspex (about 12%). Spatial resolution may be tested with a bar phantom having a range of different line pairs per millimeter. CT scanning smooths out the detail within each voxel: detail within a voxel is not imaged. Two pixels are needed to define a line pair, so resolution is about 1 lp mm^{-1}. It is much poorer than film-screen radiography.

High-resolution imaging involves increasing the matrix size or reducing the field of view, thus decreasing pixel size. Below a certain pixel size, spatial resolution is further limited by the size of the focal spot, collimators, number and size of detectors, and spacing between detectors (detail within rays being smoothed out and that between rays lost). It is also affected by patient movement.

Spatial resolution of low-contrast objects

Low-contrast spatial resolution is less good and is limited by the noise in the image. The larger the structure, the greater the number of pixels over which the noise is averaged and the better the SNR. A low-contrast structure may need to be 5–10 mm in diameter for it to be resolved.

Low-contrast spatial resolution may be assessed by imaging a slice though a Perspex phantom with water-filled holes of different diameters and different depths, thus providing different levels of contrast. Just as with an image intensifier (Fig. 4.7) a graph is plotted showing the minimum contrast needed to see, i.e. resolve, structures of different diameters. The solid curve in Fig. 4.18 shows how the spatial resolution depends on the contrast of the image, and the dashed curve shows the improvement in low-contrast perceptibility produced by increasing the mA, or dose per slice, and so reducing the noise.

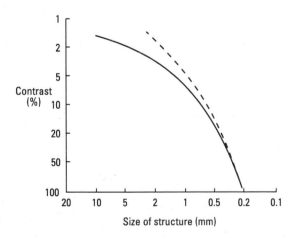

Fig. 4.18 Detail–contrast diagram for a CT scanner.

Contrast resolution

In CT, soft tissue contrast is superior to that in plain film radiography because it is not obscured by overlying bone, and scatter is smaller because of the narrow beam. Furthermore, windowing allows quite small differences of CT number to be selected from the full range and displayed over the whole grey scale.

Contrast resolution is the ability to detect small differences in the attenuation coefficient of adjacent structures. The contrast between a structure and its surroundings is only detectable if it is 3–5 times greater than the noise in the image. The more pixels a structure occupies, the less the noise and the better the contrast resolution. With a structure 10 mm in diameter, differences of 4–5 CT numbers can be detected. This is a 0.5% difference in attenuation coefficient and is at least 10 times better than can be achieved in film–screen radiography.

Resolution compromise (trade-off)

Although a spatial resolution of 1 lp mm^{-1} and a contrast resolution of 0.5% are quoted for CT, they cannot be achieved at the same time, as Fig. 4.18 makes clear. It is not possible to achieve excellent spatial and contrast resolution simultaneously, except by delivering an unacceptable dose to the patient. In fact

$$\left(\begin{array}{c}\text{slice}\\\text{thickness}\end{array}\right) \times \left(\begin{array}{c}\text{relative}\\\text{noise}\end{array}\right)^2 \times \left(\begin{array}{c}\text{pixel}\\\text{size}\end{array}\right)^3 \propto \frac{1}{\text{dose}}$$

or alternatively,

$$\left(\begin{array}{c}\text{slice}\\\text{thickness}\end{array}\right) \times \left(\begin{array}{c}\text{minimum}\\\text{detectable}\\\text{contrast}\end{array}\right)^2 \times \left(\begin{array}{c}\text{minimum}\\\text{detectable}\\\text{size}\end{array}\right)^3 \propto \frac{1}{\text{dose}}$$

Accordingly, to improve contrast detectability by a factor of 2 involves increasing the dose by a factor of 4. To improve spatial resolution by a factor of 2 involves increasing the dose by a factor of 8. To halve the slice thickness without impairing image quality involves increasing the dose by a factor of 2.

Filtering algorithms

During back-projection a 'bone' algorithm or filter may be used to enhance fine detail but at the expense of increased noise. On the other hand, a 'soft tissue' filter will improve contrast by smoothing out noise, but in doing so impairs the spatial resolution.

Dose

The distribution of absorbed dose in the body section imaged is much more uniform than in conventional radiography. With a single radiograph of the skull, if the entry skin dose is 100%, the exit skin dose might be 0.1% and the central dose 3%; in CT the skin dose is more or less uniform all round. The central dose in the head is about the same as, and in abdominal CT typically 60% of, the skin dose.

Due to scatter from one slice into adjacent slices, the dose increases somewhat with the number of slices, but not proportionally. Except that the dose is particularly high from a number of contiguous, thin (e.g. 1 mm) slices. Although the detector collimators are set to the nominal slice thickness, the actual X-ray beams overlap, as their width is much greater, being determined by the collimation near the tube.

The *CT dose index* (CTDI) is a way of gauging this spread of dose outside a nominal slice. It is the integral of the dose along the axis of the patient from a single slice divided by the nominal thickness of the slice. It can be measured by inserting a 10 cm long, thin cylindrical ionization chamber dosemeter along the axis of a cylindrical Perspex phantom and imaging one slice through its middle. Organ doses from CT examinations can be estimated by multiplying the CTDI by the appropriate conversion factors.

Typical *effective doses* are in the range 5–10 mSv per examination. Although CT scans account for only 2% of X-ray examinations, they contribute more than 20% of the radiation dose delivered to the UK population by medical X-rays.

Artefacts

Motion artefacts. Cardiac motion produces streak artefacts (black and white bands). The reconstruction process is misled by a moving structure occupying different voxels during the scan. Mechanical misalignment and movement of the patient have similar effects.

High-attenuation objects. Neurosurgical clips, dental amalgam, etc., give rise to star artefacts which may obscure the area of interest. The effect is accentuated by motion. Small areas of bone or contrast medium can have a similar effect.

Detector malfunction. In a third-generation scanner even a small imbalance in the sensitivity of the scintillation detectors can produce ring artefacts. Figure 4.19 shows how, as the gantry rotates, the X-ray pencil associated with each detector traces out a 'data ring' – a ring of tissue which is 'seen' by that detector alone. This ring can be seen on the image as an artefact if that detector malfunctions. The problem is reduced by frequent recalibration of the detectors, between patients, and is less noticeable with gas detectors, which are more easily matched.

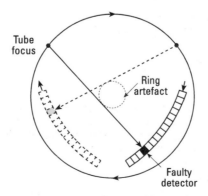

Fig. 4.19 Ring artefact associated with the third-generation scanner.

Beam hardening. The hardening of the beam which inevitably occurs as it passes through the patient causes the CT number of a given tissue to decrease along the beam path (see Section 4.3.1). The reconstruction process assumes a homogeneous X-ray beam, with the result that CT numbers are lower in the center of the patient than they should be (known as 'cupping'). This is corrected to some extent by a 'beam-hardening algorithm'.

Geometrical artefacts. Because of the diverging beam, CT slices are narrower at the center than at the edge. In consequence there may be an overlap at the edges or an unscanned region at the center.

Aliasing. A sharp and high contrast boundary (as at a bone edge) may produce a number of parallel streaks nearby in the image, for reasons explained in Section 9.2. Similarly, at the boundary between the lung and diaphragm, spurious increased density may appear in the base of the lung.

Partial volume or volume averaging artefacts. These have been described in Section 4.3.1.

Quality assurance: summary

Each department should have a quality control protocol using appropriate test objects to verify the performance of their scanners. The topics, already mentioned in this chapter include:

- *noise* – the standard deviation of the computed pixel values for the image of a water phantom, or other reference material;
- *reproducibility* – the consistency of the mean CT number for the reference material;
- *uniformity* – the variation of mean CT number over different areas of the scan field for the reference material;
- *sensitivity* – the smallest detectable object for a series of various materials (different contrasts) (see Fig. 4.18);
- *contrast scale* – the differences between the mean CT numbers for various test materials;
- *resolution* – the spatial resolution at a high contrast level;
- *alignment* – the presence or absence of streak artefacts in the scan of, for example, a high-contrast pin;
- *slice thickness* and *spacing*;
- *light beam alignment* for patient positioning;
- *dose measurements* – CTDI and dose profile.

4.3.4 Other techniques

Zoom reconstruction

An area of interest can be delineated and displayed in an enlarged format. The computed data normally used to set the grey level of one pixel on the monitor is shared between several contiguous pixels. Noise is thereby increased but resolution is effectively improved.

Scanning in other planes

Longitudinal scan. If the tube and detectors are held stationary and the couch is moved steadily along its length during the exposure, a digital image can be obtained similar to a conventional (anteroposterior, lateral, or oblique) radiographic projection. Performed at the beginning of an examination, in either the anteroposterior or lateral plane, this allows correct positioning and selection of subsequent axial images. These scout scans are produced with less patient dose than a normal radiograph.

Multiplanar imaging (sagittal, coronal, and oblique sections). A section can be taken through the three-dimensional array of CT numbers acquired with a series of separate contiguous slices and reconstructed as an image in any plane through the patient. The image so obtained has a characteristic appearance; unfortunately, the pixels are rectangular, the longer side equalling the selected slice thickness. This problem has been overcome by spiral scanning.

Spiral (helical) scanning

The couch moves continuously at a steady speed while the tube and detectors make a number of revolutions around the patient. The tube receives its power supply through slip-rings, and the detectors send their signals by radio. Suppose, for example, that the tube makes a complete rotation each second, the couch moves 10 mm s^{-1}, and the collimated slice thickness is 10 mm. In this case the pitch is 1:1 and a block of anatomy 300 mm long will be covered in 30 s, a long breath hold.

The data are *acquired* in the form of a continuous ribbon of contiguous slices, each slanted like the turns of a spiral spring. The data are *reconstructed* as a series of vertical slices, in this case 10 mm thick. Interpolation allows slices to be imaged at any level and with any incrementation. For example, a series of overlapping slices, each 10 mm thick at increments of 2 mm, could be reconstructed through a volume of interest. Note that the slice thickness cannot be changed retrospectively.

Compared with sequential CT scanning, in which the tube reverses and the patient couch is indexed between slices with separate breath holds, spiral scanning has the following advantages and disadvantages:

◆ *Advantages*. It is faster, thus allowing a greater throughput of patients and also the use of a smaller volume of contrast medium. (A double-helical scanner with two rows of detectors is even faster.) It overcomes the problem of slice-to-slice misregistration, particularly in the region of the diaphragm, caused by variations in inspiration between the separate breath holds needed in sequential scanning. It reduces partial volume artefacts since the reconstructed slices can be incremented in small steps. Because of the volume acquisition of data, resolution in the axial direction is good, and reformatting into other planes is improved.

◆ *Disadvantages*. There being no cooling periods between slices, the heat loading of the tube is high. Even though a high-capacity tube and sensitive detectors are used, a lower mA must be employed. As a result, patient dose may be lower but noise may be greater, particularly with thicker patients. There may also be some loss of spatial resolution due to the interpolation process. A high-speed computer with a large data store is necessary.,

Pitch is defined as the distance (millimeters) moved by the table during one rotation of the tube divided by the slice thickness (millimeters). Increasing the pitch, by increasing the table speed, is like stretching the spring; it speeds up scanning, reduces dose, but resolution may be lost through the greater interpolation needed. Above a pitch of 2:1 there are gaps in the volume being scanned, and artefacts may arise.

Two-dimensional reformatting

Imaginary, mathematical, parallel 'rays' may be sent in any chosen direction through the three-dimensional array of CT data in the computer memory, and projected on to a selected image plane. As each ray encounters the CT numbers in the voxels it passes through, it may first reject the high numbers corresponding to bone if it is required to remove bone from the image. Then:

(a) In *shaded surface display* (SSD) any CT number so encountered in any voxel along each ray is recorded in a corresponding pixel in the image plane, provided it exceeds a set threshold value. The image is displayed as if illuminated by an imaginary light source, and is particularly useful in plastic surgery.

(b) In *maximum intensity projection* (MIP) the highest CT number so encountered in any voxel along each ray is recorded in a corresponding pixel in the image plane. Calcified lesions and contrast media can be distinguished. These procedures find particular application in CT angiography and arthrography.

Three-dimensional reformatting

Multiple projections may be made in this way, around an axis of rotation, and displayed in a cine loop as a rotating three-dimensional representation of anatomy, either as a shaded surface image or a volume rendered (see-through) display. These software manipulations are very computer-hungry and may be time-consuming.

Cine computed tomography scanning

A continuously rotating scanner can also be used with the couch stationary to take a sequence of images of a single slice, e.g. to study the passage of contrast medium through the slice and to allow the best image to be selected for interpretation.

4.4 PICTURE ARCHIVING AND COMMUNICATION SYSTEM (PACS)

As described in later chapters, digital images are produced in gamma imaging, position emission tomography, single-photon emission CT, ultrasound scanning, and magnetic resonance imaging, as well as in digital fluoroscopy and CT. In addition, conventional radiographs can be digitized by special laser beam scanners. To match the definition of the radiograph a 2048^2 matrix, 2 bytes deep, would be necessary.

These sources of digital information can be networked, within a department or hospital, with a central computer and video monitors in clinics, wards, etc. Computing techniques can be used to increase information. Vascular structures can be enhanced by subtraction; fractures by edge enhancement; and soft tissue contrast by windowing. Images can be panned, zoomed, and scrolled. With care, images produced by different modalities can be registered and superimposed. High-resolution anatomical images (CT and magnetic resonance imaging) can be overlaid with low-resolution functional images (positron emission tomography and single-photon emission CT).

Images can be archived compactly in a 'juke box' of optical disks, totalling 1 terabyte, say, and rapidly accessed from the peripheral video consoles, and hard copies produced when needed using a laser camera. A PACS can be integrated with the department's reporting system and the hospital's computerized information system, including the laboratories. Digital images can also be transmitted to other hospitals. Computer-assisted image evaluation and diagnosis are the subjects of current research.

Silverless radiography

Silverless imaging departments have become a reality, eliminating the need for any wet processing and saving on a relatively scarce and costly natural resource. A conventional film may be substituted by a flexible polyester base on which is coated a photostimulable phosphor (see Section 1.7) such as europium-activated barium fluorohalide. It is loaded into a cassette and exposed in the usual way. Half of the X-ray energy absorbed by the phosphor is immediately emitted as fluorescent light, which is wasted. The other half is stored as trapped electrons.

The plate carries a latent image of stored energy which is released by scanning it rasterwise with a very narrow beam of light from a helium–neon laser. The light emitted is measured by a photomultiplier. The digitized signal is handled and displayed as in other forms of digital imaging. A computer can be used to enhance either the contrast or spatial resolution, whichever is appropriate to the site being examined. The plate is exposed to a bright light before reuse.

A particular advantage of the system is its wide latitude. It is linear over a 10 000:1 range of X-ray intensities compared to the 100:1 range over which the characteristic curve of a film is linear. Images of similar quality (spatial and contrast resolution) to a fast film-screen can be obtained with about half the dose.

It would be appropriate at this point to read Chapter 9, which develops further some of the ideas encountered in this chapter and shows how they apply to the other forms of imaging described in later chapters.

4.5 APPENDIX

Whereas decimal numbers are based on powers of 10, *binary numbers* are based on powers of two. (Within a computer a voltage of 0 V represents the digit 0 and a voltage e.g. 5 V represents the digit 1.) The 10-bit binary number 10101 01010, for example, stands for

$$(1 \times 512) + (0 \times 256) + (1 \times 128) + (0 \times 64) + (1 \times 32) +$$
$$(0 \times 16) + (1 \times 8) + (0 \times 4) + (1 \times 2) + (0 \times 1) = 682.$$

A 10-bit number can have any one of $2^{10} = 1024$ values between 1 and 1023, and can represent any one of 1024 different grey levels in an image. A byte (B) = 8 bits; 1 kilobyte (kB) = 1024 bytes; similarly with megabyte (MB), gigabyte (GB), and terabyte (TB).

VIVA QUESTIONS

1. How does an image intensifier work?

2. What is an input (output) phosphor and how does it work?

3. In what kinds of equipment do you find photomultipliers?

4. How does a photomultiplier function?

5. Why may a partial mirror be used in a fluoroscopic system?

6. What is the difference in dose rate at the image intensifier between cineradiography at 35 frames s^{-1} and videotaping of the same image?

7. What is meant by the term 'spatial resolution'?

8. How is spatial resolution measured in relation to (a) fluoroscopy, (b) computed tomography, and (c) conventional radiography; and what are the differences between them?

9. In relation to a TV monitor, what is meant by (a) contrast resolution, (b) lag, and (c) dynamic range or latitude?

10. What types of CT scanner do you know? Explain the operation of the different generations of scanner.

11. What are the principles behind CT?

12. Compare and contrast the different detectors used in CT.

13. What is a Hounsfield number?

14. What are meant by the terms 'window width' and 'window level'?

15. Compare the dose to the patient from CT scans with conventional radiographic films, such as a chest X-ray.

16. Name and describe some artefacts related to CT scanning.

17. How does spiral CT differ from a conventional CT scanner?

18. Explain the importance of signal-to-noise ratios in CT scanning.

19. What factors can you adjust on CT scanners to improve the signal-to-noise ratio?

20. What routine tests would you carry out on your CT scanner to assure the image quality?

GAMMA IMAGING

5.1 RADIOACTIVITY

Stable nuclei

Nearly all the nuclides extant in the world are stable. Apart from the nucleus of ordinary hydrogen, which consists of a single proton, all the stable lighter nuclei contain nearly equal numbers of protons and neutrons. For example, the nucleus of a helium atom (otherwise known as an alpha particle) is a very stable combination of two neutrons and two protons. The heavier nuclei contain a greater proportion of neutrons.

Isotopes

The nuclei of all carbon atoms contain six protons. Ninety-nine percent of stable carbon nuclei are carbon-12 (^{12}C) with six neutrons; 1% are carbon-13 (^{13}C) with seven neutrons. Carbon-11 (^{11}C) with only five neutrons has a neutron deficit, and carbon-14 (^{14}C) with eight neutrons has a neutron excess; both are artificially produced, unstable, and radioactive. All four nuclides are isotopes of carbon.

Isotopes of an element are nuclides which have the *same* number of protons, atomic number, position in the periodic table, and chemical and metabolic properties, but a *different* number of neutrons, mass number, density, and other physical properties.

Radionuclides

Unstable nuclei, having a neutron excess or deficit, are radioactive and transform spontaneously (or 'decay') until they become stable nuclei, with the emission of any combination of alpha, beta, and gamma radiation.

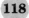

Production of radionuclides. There are a few radionuclides which are sufficiently long lived to occur in nature, e.g. uranium, radium, and radon. However, those used in medical imaging must be produced artificially, in the following ways:

◈ If an additional neutron is forced into a stable nucleus, so that it now has a *neutron excess*, the new nucleus is likely to be unstable. This process occurs in a *nuclear reactor*, e.g. with molybdenum (Mo):

$$^{98}\text{Mo} + \text{n} \rightarrow {}^{99}\text{Mo}$$

The atomic number of the nucleus remains unchanged but its mass number has increased by one. Radionuclides produced in a nuclear reactor cannot be separated from the original stable nuclides as they have the same atomic number and so the same chemical properties. They cannot be made 'carrier-free'.

◈ If an additional proton is forced into a stable nucleus knocking out a neutron, so that it now has a *neutron deficit*, the new nucleus is likely to be unstable. For example, with boron:

$$^{11}\text{B} + \text{p} \rightarrow {}^{11}\text{C} + \text{n}$$

The mass number of the nucleus has not changed but its atomic number has increased by one. This process occurs in a *cyclotron* which accelerates positively charged ions: protons, deuterons, or alpha particles.

Radionuclides produced in a cyclotron can be obtained carrier-free. They can be separated chemically from the original stable nuclides as they have different atomic numbers and so different chemical properties. They are also short lived, and so it is only possible to use them reasonably near to the cyclotron.

◈ Radioactive *fission products* may be extracted from the spent fuel rods of nuclear reactors.

◈ In addition to the nuclear reactor and the cyclotron, some radionuclides are obtained from *generators* (see Section 5.5)

5.2 RADIOACTIVE TRANSFORMATION (DECAY)

Nuclides with a neutron excess: β^- decay

Such nuclides may lose energy and become stable by a neutron changing into a proton and an electron. The electron is ejected from the nucleus with high energy, and is referred to as a negative beta particle:

$$\text{n} \rightarrow \text{p} + \beta^-$$

For example, iodine-131 (^{131}I) with atomic number 53 decays in this way to xenon-31 (^{131}Xe) with atomic number 54. There has been no change of mass number but the atomic number has increased by one. Nearly always the product or daughter nucleus is produced with excess energy. Usually it loses this immediately, with the emission of one or more gamma photons, leaving the daughter nucleus with minimum energy, in the 'ground state'.

Isomeric transition (IT). In the case of some radionuclides the gamma ray is not emitted until an appreciable time after the emission of the beta particle. For example, when molybdenum-99 (^{99}Mo) decays by the emission of a negative beta particle, the daughter nucleus technetium-99 (^{99}Tc)

remains in the excited state for a variable length of time, which averages a matter of hours. It is said to be metastable, and is written technetium-99m or ^{99m}Tc. This decays rather quickly to the ground state ^{99}Tc, most often with the emission of a gamma ray of energy 140 keV.

$$^{99}_{42}\text{Mo} \xrightarrow[67\,\text{h}]{\beta^-,\gamma} {}^{99m}_{43}\text{Tc} \xrightarrow[6\,\text{h}]{\gamma} {}^{99}_{43}\text{Tc} \xrightarrow[0.2\,\text{Ma}]{\beta^-,\gamma} \text{stable nuclide}$$

Note the convention used:

$$\text{parent nuclide} \xrightarrow[\text{half-life}]{\text{emission}} \text{daughter nuclide}$$

^{99m}Tc and ^{99}Tc are said to be isomers: nuclei having different energy states but otherwise indistinguishable as regards mass number, atomic number, numbers of protons, and neutrons and other properties.

Whereas ^{99}Mo emits both beta and gamma rays; ^{99m}Tc emits gamma rays only. The transformation

$$^{99m}\text{Tc} \rightarrow {}^{99}\text{Tc} + \gamma$$

is an isomeric transition.

Another isomeric transition used in nuclear imaging occurs when rubidium-81 (^{81}Rb) decays to krypton-81 (^{81}Kr)

$$^{81}\text{Rb} \rightarrow {}^{81m}\text{Kr} \rightarrow {}^{81}\text{Kr}$$

Nuclides with a neutron deficit

β^+ decay. Such nuclides may lose energy and become stable by a proton within the nucleus changing into a neutron and a positive electron. The latter is ejected from the nucleus with high energy, and is referred to as a positive beta particle. Mass and charge are conserved:

$$p \rightarrow n + \beta^+$$

For example, ^{11}C with atomic number 6 transforms into boron-11 (^{11}B) with atomic number 5. There has been no change of mass number but the atomic number has decreased by one. The product or daughter nucleus, if left in an excited state, loses its excess energy by the emission of one or more gamma photons until it reaches the ground state.

K-electron capture (EC)

Alternatively, the nucleus may increase its number of neutrons relative to the number of protons by capturing an extranuclear electron from the nearest (K) shell. Mass and charge are again conserved:

$$p + e^- \rightarrow n$$

The daughter nuclide will emit characteristic X-rays when the hole so created in the K-shell is filled by an electron from an outer shell. If the daughter nuclide is left in an excited state it will also emit gamma rays. For example, iodine-123 (^{123}I) decays wholly by electron capture and emits 160 keV gamma and 28 keV X-rays, but no beta particles.

Gamma rays

The gamma ray emitted during radioactive decay of a given radionuclide have at most a few specific energies (forming a line spectrum) which are characteristic of the nuclide which emits them. For example, ^{131}I emits mostly 360 keV gamma rays. Gamma rays have identical properties to X-rays, as described in Chapter 1.

Internal conversion (IC). The gamma rays emitted by some nuclei do not leave the atom, but are photoelectrically absorbed in its K-shell. As a result of this internal conversion, such radionuclides emit both photoelectrons and characteristic X-rays, usually of fairly low energy.

Beta rays

The beta rays are emitted with a continuous spectrum of energies up to a maximum E_{max} which is characteristic of the radionuclide. Their average energy is about $E_{max}/3$. When positive and negative beta particles travel through a material, being moving electrons they interact with the outer shells of the atoms they pass nearby and excite and ionize them. The track of the particle is dotted with ion pairs. When it has lost the whole of its initial energy it comes to the end of its range. The greater the initial energy of the beta particle, the greater its range. The range is inversely proportional to the density of the material. The most energetic beta rays have a range of about 2 mm in tissue, but those produced by most radionuclides have a much shorter range.

Positron emitters

Positive electrons, being antimatter, have a very brief existence. When a positive beta particle comes to the end of its range it combines with a nearby negative electron. The opposite charges neutralize each other, and the combined masses of the two electrons are wholly converted into energy. According to Einstein's formula ($E = mc^2$) for the equivalence between energy E and mass m, the mass of each electron is equivalent to 511 keV. When the positive and negative electrons annihilate each other, the energy is emitted as two photons of annihilation radiation (each of 511 keV) traveling in opposite directions. Positron emitters are used in positron emission tomography (PET) imaging (see Section 5.8.2).

Radioactive decay

Radioactive disintegration is a stochastic process, governed by the statistical laws of chance. It is impossible to predict which of the unstable nuclei in a sample will disintegrate in the next second, but it is possible to be quite precise about the fraction that will do so, on account of the large numbers of nuclei the sample contains.

Activity. A radioactive nucleus does not make its presence known until it decays and emits a beta or a gamma ray, or both. The quantity of radioactivity is measured not by the 'population', the mass or number of radioactive atoms, but by the 'death rate', the transformation rate, the number which disintegrate per second.

The activity of a radioactive sample is the rate of disintegration: the number of nuclei disintegrating per second. The SI unit is the becquerel (Bq) = 1 disintegration per second. This is a very low activity: the natural radioactive content of the human body is about 2 kBq (2000 Bq). In imaging, most radionuclide administrations are measured in megabecquerels (1 MBq = 10^6 Bq), and the activity of radionuclide generators in gigabecquerels (1 GBq = 10^9 Bq). (An older unit is the curie (Ci); 1 mCi = 37 MBq.)

When the beta or gamma rays enter a detector they may be registered individually as 'counts'. The count rate (number of counts per second, cps) measured by a given instrument is less than the activity because the greater proportion of the rays usually miss the detector and some pass through it undetected. However,

Count rate ∝ activity ∝ number or mass of radioactive atoms in the sample

The fundamental *law of radioactive decay* states that the activity of a radioactive sample decreases by equal fractions (percentages) in equal intervals of time. This is referred to as the exponential law.

Physical half-life.   The half-life ($t_{1/2}$) of a radionuclide is the time taken for its activity to decay to half of its original value. For example, two successive half-lives reduce the activity of a radionuclide by a factor of $2 \times 2 = 4$. Ten half-lives reduce the activity by a factor of $2^{10} \approx 1000$.

This half-life is more properly called the physical half-life. It is a fixed characteristic of the radionuclide, cannot be predicted in any way, and is unaffected by any agency such as heat, pressure, electricity, or chemical reactions. It can range from fractions of a second (useless in imaging) to millennia in the case of ^{99}Tc (also useless in imaging). Examples are given in Table 5.1.

Exponential decay.   However long the time, the activity of a radioactive sample never falls to zero. This is shown by the shape – an exponential curve – of the graph of activity versus time, both being plotted on linear scales. If, however, the activity is plotted on a logarithmic scale, a straight-line graph results (Fig. 5.1), making it easier to read off the half-life.

Table 5.1 Half-lives of radionuclides

Half-life	Nuclide
13 s	Krypton-81m
1 min	Rubidium-82
10 min	Nitrogen-13
20 min	Carbon-11
68 min	Gallium-68
112 min	Fluorine-18
6 h	Technetium-99m
13 h	Iodine-123
67 h	Molybdenum-99
67 h	Indium-111
73 h	Thallium-201
78 h	Gallium-67
5 days	Xenon-133
8 days	Iodine-131
200 000 years	Technetium-99

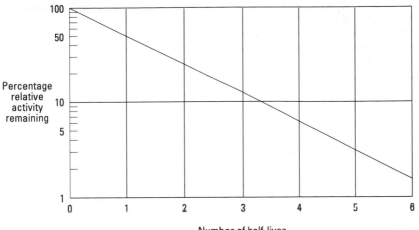

Fig. 5.1 Exponential decay. Activity on a logarithmic scale against time on a linear scale.

Such graphs are useful in calculating (a) the activity which must be prepared at a particular time for use at a subsequent time and (b) how long it is necessary to store radioactivity before it becomes sufficiently harmless to be disposed of safely.

Effective half-life. When a radionuclide is used in imaging it usually forms part of a salt or organic compound, the metabolic properties of which ensure that it concentrates in the tissues or organ of interest. The pharmaceutical has been 'labeled' with the radionuclide.

If the pharmaceutical alone is administered it is gradually eliminated from the tissues, organ, and whole body by the usual metabolic processes of turnover and excretion. Such a process can be regarded as having a biological half-life t_{biol}.

If the radionuclide is stored in a bottle, its activity decays with its physical half-life t_{phys}.

If the labeled radiopharmaceutical is administered to a person, the activity in specific tissues, an organ, or the whole body decreases due to the simultaneous effects of (a) radioactive decay and (b) metabolic turnover and excretion. The activity can be regarded as having an effective half-life t_{eff}.

The effective half-life is shorter than either the biological or physical half-lives. In fact

$$1/t_{eff} = 1/t_{biol} + 1/t_{phys}$$

It depends on the radiopharmaceutical used and the organ, etc., involved, and can vary from person to person, depending on their disease state.

5.3 GAMMA IMAGING

The patient is given an appropriate radiopharmaceutical, usually by intravenous injection. The function of the pharmaceutical is, ideally, to concentrate in the organ or tissues of interest. The role of the radionuclide is to signal the location of the radiopharmaceutical by the emission of gamma rays. The radionuclide most commonly used, ^{99m}Tc, emits 140 keV gamma rays. These are collected by a gamma camera, and an image of the radioactive distribution is produced on a monitor screen. Since gamma rays cannot be focused, instead of a lens a multihole collimator is used to delineate the image from the patient.

A gamma camera has heavy lead shielding to attenuate unwanted background gamma radiation coming from the patient generally, any other sources in the room, and building materials.

The multihole collimator

The patient is positioned, as shown in Fig. 5.2, close to the collimator. This consists of a lead disk, typically 25 mm thick and up to 400 mm in diameter. It is drilled with some 20 000 closely packed circular or hexagonal holes, each 2.5 mm in diameter. They are separated by septa 0.3 mm thick which absorb all but a few percent of the rays attempting to pass through them obliquely. (The half value layer (HVL) of lead for ^{99m}Tc gamma rays is 0.3 mm.)

Each hole only accepts gamma rays from a narrow channel, thus locating any radioactive source along its line of sight. For example, in Fig. 5.2, ray a is accepted by the collimator, and ray b rejected. However, other rays such as c can be scattered in the body and then pass through the collimator. These rays will have less energy and so can be rejected later by energy discrimination (see 'pulse height analyzer', below).

The crystal

Instead of an equally large number of tiny detectors, behind the collimator there lies a single large phosphor crystal some 500 mm in diameter and 9–12 mm thick, made of sodium iodide (activated with a trace of thallium). Having a high atomic number ($Z = 53$) and density, it absorbs about 90% of ^{99m}Tc gamma rays, principally by the photoelectric process; but only some 30% of those from ^{131}I. It is fragile and easily damaged by temperature changes. To protect it from light and the atmosphere (it is hygroscopic) it is encapsulated in an aluminum cylinder with one flat Pyrex face.

Each gamma photon (such as photon a in Fig. 5.2) when absorbed by the crystal produces a flash of light, shown by the dashed lines in the diagram. The flash contains some 5000 light photons which travel in all directions and last less than a microsecond. About 4000 of them emerge from the farther flat surface, having been reflected off the other faces, which are coated with a reflecting titanium compound. The distribution of light leaving the face of the crystal depends upon which collimator hole the gamma ray passed through, and is measured by up to 91 matched photomultipliers, closely packed in a hexagonal array. Five of these are shown, diagrammatically, in Fig. 5.2. Transfer of light from the crystal to the photomultipliers may be maximized by a light guide – a flat transparent plate.

Photomultipliers

Each photomultiplier (Fig. 5.3) consists of an evacuated glass envelope containing (on the left) a photocathode coated with a material which absorbs light and emits photoelectrons: one electron per five or 10 light

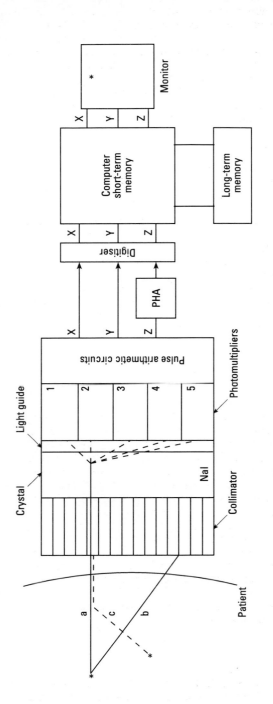

Fig. 5.2 Schematic diagram of a gamma camera. (PHA, pulse height analyzer.)

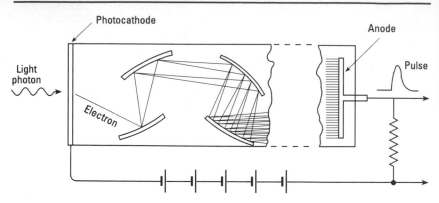

Fig. 5.3 Photomultiplier tube.

photons. These are accelerated toward a positive anode (on the right). *En route* they impinge on a series of dynodes which are connected to progressively increasing positive potentials. Four such dynodes are depicted in the diagram.

When each electron strikes a dynode it knocks out some 3–4 electrons, which are then accelerated, as shown, to strike the next dynode. In this, way, after 10 stages, the electrons have been multiplied by a factor $4^{10}=10^6$. Thus each initial flash of light produces a pulse of charge or voltage large enough to be measured electronically. The amplification factor is very sensitive to changes in the overall voltage (about 1 kV), which has to be highly stabilized.

Pulse arithmetic (position logic)

Returning to Fig. 5.2, the light pulse illuminates differentially the array of photomultiplier tubes. It produces the largest electrical pulse in the photomultiplier (No. 2) nearest to the collimator hole through which the gamma ray a passed – and smaller pulses in adjacent photomultipliers. A microprocessor chip, the 'pulse arithmetic circuit', combines the pulses from all the photomultipliers according to certain equations. This yields three voltage pulses (X, Y, Z) which are proportional to:

◆ The horizontal or X and vertical or Y coordinates of the light flash in the crystal, the hole through which the gamma ray has passed, and so the position in the body of the radioactive atom that has emitted it (X, Y).

◆ The photon energy of the original gamma ray (Z). For this purpose the pulses from all the photomultipliers are simply summed, as if there were one large photomultiplier, measuring all the light produced by the gamma ray in the phosphor crystal. The size or 'height' of the Z-pulse (so many volts) is proportional to the gamma ray energy (in kiloelectronvolts) absorbed. For convenience the pulse height is generally stated in the corresponding kiloelectronvolts.

Pulse height spectrum

The account so far ignores two facts:

◆ gamma rays are scattered in the patient, so that gamma rays which

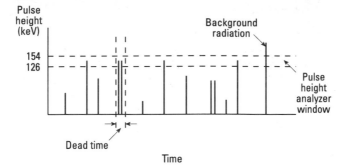

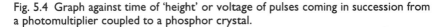

Fig. 5.4 Graph against time of 'height' or voltage of pulses coming in succession from a photomultiplier coupled to a phosphor crystal.

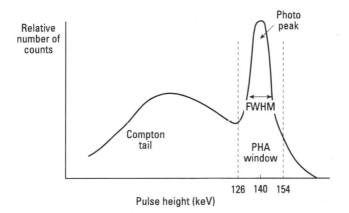

Fig. 5.5 A pulse height spectrum showing the relative frequency of pulses of various heights, (FWHM, full width at half maximum. PHA, pulse height analyzer.)

have originated outside the line of sight of the collimator can enter a collimator hole, and, as they have been scattered, do so with reduced energy (ray c in Fig. 5.2);

◈ gamma rays may lose energy through Compton interactions in the crystal before being absorbed photoelectrically, and so produce only pulses of reduced height.

When a large number of gamma rays are emitted in succession within a patient the Z-pulses therefore vary in height. Taking 99mTc as an example, Fig. 5.4 illustrates a sequence of such pulses; it plots the pulse height (kiloelectronvolts) against time. Figure 5.5 plots the relative number of pulses having various heights or energies, in a given period of time. This pulse height spectrum is made up of:

◈ A *photopeak*, on the right, comprising pulses produced by the complete photoelectric absorption in the crystal of those gamma ray photons which have come from within the patient without suffering Compton scattering.

They vary somewhat in height, lying within a 'window' shown by the horizontal dashed lines in Fig. 5.4.

The spread of energies in the photopeak, evident in Fig. 5.5, is due to statistical fluctuations in both (a) the number of light photons produced in the crystal by each gamma ray photon and (b) the number of electrons produced in the photomultiplier by each light photon. This also causes the short tail on the right.

◆ A *tail*, on the left, containing pulses of lower energy, mostly produced by those gamma rays which have suffered Compton interactions in either the patient or the crystal. (There is also a subsidiary 'iodine escape peak' at 30 keV below the photopeak, due to some of the K-characteristic rays from iodine escaping from the crystal.) Only pulses in the photopeak are of use in locating the source of the radioactivity in the patient, and a pulse height analyzer is used to reject those in the Compton tail

Pulse height analyzer

As shown in Fig. 5.2, the Z-pulses enter a pulse height analyzer, which is set by the operator to reject pulses which are either (a) lower than a preset value or (b) higher than another preset value. It lets through only those pulses which lie within a window of, say, ±10% of the photopeak energy. The pulses so selected are referred to as 'counts'. As Fig. 5.4 illustrates, any high-energy background radiation is also rejected.

In the case of ^{99m}Tc the window might be set at 126–154 keV, centered on 140 keV (Fig. 5.5). Even so, because a 140 keV photon will lose only 10 keV of energy even when scattered through 45°, some scattered photons may 'pass through' the window, produce counts, and so degrade the image. In the case of ^{67}Ga or ^{111}In, two or three windows must be used simultaneously, each selecting one gamma ray energy.

The X-, Y-, and Z-pulses are next applied, as shown in Fig. 5.2, either (a) directly to a monitor for visual interpretation, as in older machines, or (b) in newer systems via analog-to-digital converters (ADCs) into a computer. This enables dynamic and gated studies to be undertaken as well as a range of image processing.

The monitor

The X- and Y-pulses steer the electron beam in the monitor tube. If and only if the Z-pulse has passed through the window of the pulse height analyzer does a pinpoint of light appear momentarily on the screen (see Fig. 5.2) at the X- and Y-coordinates corresponding to the heights of the X- and Y-pulses and the positions of the radioactive atom emitting each gamma ray. Thousands of such dots, equally bright, make up the image. Two types of monitor are used:

◆ a *long persistence screen* on which each dot of light persists for a sufficiently long time for a visual image to build up of the radioactivity in the patient. The image quality is not good enough for diagnosis but is helpful for positioning the patient and making sure that the activity has been taken up.

◆ a *short persistence screen* of high quality, on which each dot quickly dies away but can be captured on film, in a camera, on which an image of the radioactivity in the patient gradually builds up.

Either a polaroid or a multiformat film *camera* can be used. The latter employs single-coated cut transparency film, formulated for an X-ray automatic processor. If required, a number of images can be recorded in sequence side by side on a single film. Polaroid film has high speed and resolution and can be processed very quickly. It is, however, expensive, and has a low contrast and a limited dynamic range.

If the film is exposed for too long, it will be saturated; if for too short a time, the image will be underexposed, faint, and grainy. Typically, a total of 0.5 million counts is acquired for each image, taking about 5 min.

The computer

After digitization with an ADC, the X-, Y- and Z-pulses pass to a computer which records each Z-pulse as a count in a memory location corresponding to the X- and Y-coordinates. As the pulses arrive at random, the counts build up in each location and are stored as a digital image in a 128×128 matrix. When complete, it is scanned by a television raster and displayed on a monitor screen as a 128×128 matrix of 3 mm pixels. The brightness of each pixel depends on the number of counts stored in the corresponding memory location, i.e. to the number of gamma rays which have emanated from the corresponding area of the patient and to the activity therein.

If counts were acquired for too long, the memory locations would become full (an 8-bit memory can hold 2^8 counts) and the monitor screen would become more or less uniformly bright. If they were acquired for too short a time the image would be grainy. Typically, a total of 500 000 or 1 million counts are acquired for each image frame.

Before display, the stored image can be manipulated and improved in the usual ways, described in Chapter 4. Background can be suppressed, blurring reduced, contrast enhanced by windowing, noise reduced by averaging, and the matrix increased and made less evident by pixel interpolation. Quantitative data can be extracted, e.g. a plot of activity along a selected line. Separate images of two radionuclides, administered at the same time, can be obtained with different settings of the pulse height analyzer. If desired, one image can be subtracted, pixel by pixel, from the other.

Dynamic imaging

The function of kidney, lungs, heart, etc., can be studied by acquiring a series of separate images (frames) in suitably rapid succession. The images can be retrieved from the computer store in sequence and either (a) recorded side by side on a single film in a multiformat camera or (b) repeatedly displayed *seriatim* on the screen as a cine loop.

Areas of interest (e.g. kidneys) can be defined by cursors, and the total counts therein measured on each frame and displayed as a function of time (e.g. a renogram). An area of interest can be defined between the kidneys and used for background subtraction.

In multiple-gated cardiac studies, separate frames, each lasting 40 ms, are acquired at 20–30 different points in each cardiac cycle. At each such point, several hundred successive images are added, pixel by pixel, to improve statistics and so reduce noise. Each sequence is initiated by the R-wave from an electrocardiogram. The images can be recorded separately in a multiformat mode or displayed as a cine loop of the pulsating heart. Quantitative data about heart function can be extracted.

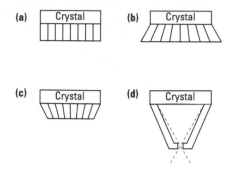

Fig. 5.6 Types of collimator, (a) Parallel hole, (b) divergent hole, (c) convergent hole, and (d) pinhole.

Collimators

Most commonly used with a 400 mm camera is the parallel hole collimator (Fig. 5.6a). The field of view and the sensitivity are the same at all distances from the collimator face.

With a smaller diameter camera, a larger field of view can be obtained by a divergent hole collimator (Fig. 5.6b), which minifies the image, allowing a large organ such as the lung to be imaged with a small crystal such as in a mobile gamma camera. A convergent hole collimator (Fig. 5.6c), in which the holes converge to a point in the patient, magnifies the image but reduces the field of view, and may be useful when imaging children. Resolution deteriorates toward the edge of the field.

Both of these special collimators suffer from geometrical distortion: the back of an organ is magnified differently from the front; and the field of view and sensitivity both vary with distance.

A pinhole collimator (Fig. 5.6d), a cone of lead with a single hole a few millimeters in diameter at its apex, can be used to produce a magnified but inverted image of a superficial small organ such as the thyroid.

The sensitivity of a collimator measures the proportion of gamma rays, falling on it from all directions, that pass through the holes. It is only a fraction of a percent. The more holes there are, or the wider they are or the shorter they are, the greater the sensitivity, the less radionuclide needs to be administered, and so the less the patient dose.

Spatial resolution. Figure 5.7 illustrates one of the holes in a collimator, lying between the crystal and the surface of the patient. Gamma rays originating anywhere between the inner dotted lines 'illuminate' the whole of the 'visible' crystal surface and produce a maximum signal. Gamma rays originating anywhere outside the outer dashed lines are cut off by the lead septa and produce no signal. Gamma rays originating from any points along the solid lines illuminate exactly half of the crystal face. R is the spatial resolution of the collimator. It is larger, i.e. worse, when the distance from the face of the collimator is increased. It is best close to the collimator, and the patient should be positioned accordingly.

The wider the holes or the shorter they are, the greater the sensitivity but the worse the spatial resolution. It follows that the better the resolution, the less the sensitivity. It is not possible to maximize both

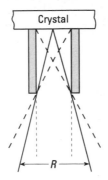

Fig. 5.7 Spatial resolution of a single-hole collimator.

sensitivity and spatial resolution, and a compromise must be made. This is a major limitation to the performance of a gamma camera.

Types of collimator. *Low energy collimators* have thin septa (0.3 mm) and can be used with gamma rays of up to 150 keV, e.g. with 99mTc. A *general-purpose* collimator might have 20 000 holes each 2.5 mm diameter, a resolution (10 cm from the face) of 9 mm, and sensitivity 150 cps MBq^{-1}. A *high-resolution* collimator would have more and smaller holes and lower sensitivity. It can be used where high resolution is required and the amount of radioactivity and the imaging times needed are acceptable. A *high-sensitivity* collimator would have fewer and larger holes and poorer resolution. It can be used in dynamic imaging where short exposure times are necessary and the poorer resolution must be accepted.

Medium-energy collimators, for use up to 400 keV, e.g. with 111In, 67Ga, and 131I, have thicker septa (1.4 mm) and consequently fewer holes and lower sensitivity.

Types of gamma camera

The 400 mm general-purpose camera described above is optimized for 99mTc. A mobile gamma camera is designed for cardiac imaging. It has a 250 mm field and a crystal 5 mm thick which gives good resolution with the 80 keV gamma rays from 201Tl. Being easy to position, it is used in cardiac stress laboratories and intensive care units.

A large field of view (500 mm) camera can take in the whole width of the patient and is used in bone and gallium imaging. A scanning gamma camera, in which the head translates along the patient, effectively increases the image matrix from 128 × 128 to 128 × 512.

5.4 CHARACTERISTICS AND QUALITY ASSURANCE OF THE GAMMA IMAGE

Uniformity of field

A flood field phantom consists of a flat sealed dish, larger than the field of view (FOV), filled with 99mTc or its longer lived analog cobalt-57

(^{57}Co). This should give a uniform image both with and without the collimator in place: a defective photomultiplier will be seen as a dark area in the image. A cracked crystal will show as a linear defect. Nonuniformity due to slight differences in the performance of individual photomultipliers is assessed by instructing the computer to compute a histogram of the counts in individual pixels. (A sufficiently long exposure is necessary to reduce noise.) It calculates the standard deviation and the mean. Typically the uniformity is 1 or 2%. Modern gamma cameras, when presented with a flood field phantom, can be instructed to compensate subsequent images automatically for minor nonuniformities of the field.

Spatial resolution

This is the ability of the system to produce distinct images of two small radioactive sources close together.

Intrinsic resolution. This refers to the camera (crystal, photomultipliers, and position logic circuits) in the absence of the collimator and patient. When a single gamma photon is absorbed at a point in the crystal, the 4000 or so photons of emerging light only eject a total of 400 or so electrons from the photocathodes of all the photomultipliers. In Fig. 5.2, photomultipliers Nos. 1 and 3 should receive equal numbers of photons and produce identical pulses. However, on account of the small numbers of light photons and electrons involved, there are significant statistical variations in the relative numbers and a difference in the heights of the pulses they produce. This leads to errors in the X- and Y-coordinates assigned to the event, and so causes blurring of the image. Intrinsic resolution can be improved by using a thinner crystal but with consequent reduction in sensitivity (just as with intensifying screens).

System resolution. The intrinsic blurring is compounded (according to the same formula as for radiographic blurrings) by the additional blurring caused by (a) the collimator and (b) scattering of gamma rays in the patient. Resolution worsens the farther the activity is from the collimator. Consequently it is worse for fat patients than for thin.

Testing the resolution. Resolution can be tested by imaging a line source. The computer is instructed to plot the counts along a line of pixels at right angles to a thin tube filled with ^{99m}Tc. The graph (Fig. 5.8) is called the '*line spread function*'.

The line source can be placed:

◆ Against the face of the collimator in air (solid curve). The spread of the curve (measured halfway up, called the 'full width to half maximum' or FWHM) corresponds to R in Fig. 5.7, and is typically 5 mm.

◆ Against the crystal face after removing the collimator (dotted curve). The FWHM of this curve measures the intrinsic resolution, typically between 1 and 2 mm for a modern camera.

◆ At 10 cm deep in a scattering medium while using the collimator, for system resolution (dashed curve). (This depth is chosen, as the organs being imaged typically lie between 5 and 10 cm deep.) The FWHM of this curve measures the system resolution, typically 10 mm. Resolution is

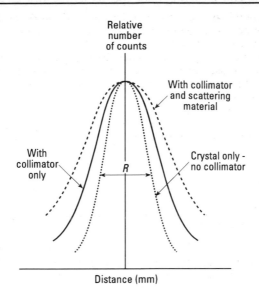

Fig. 5.8 Spatial resolution of a gamma camera.

therefore not improved by using a smaller pixel size than 3 mm in a 128 × 128 matrix.

Alternatively, spatial resolution can be tested with a bar test pattern – made of either strips of lead placed on a flood field phantom or evenly spaced parallel line sources – placed against the face of the crystal. This measures the intrinsic resolution, typically 3–6 lp cm^{-1}. In practice the overall system resolution is worse than 1 lp cm^{-1}, and the value of gamma imaging lies in evaluating function rather than anatomy.

Linearity

Linearity (i.e. lack of distortion) can also be checked by imaging a line source.

Energy resolution

This is the ability to distinguish between separate gamma rays of different energies. Its importance lies in the fact that the better the energy resolution, the better the rejection of scatter and the better the spatial resolution.

As remarked earlier, when a single gamma photon is absorbed by a crystal, the resulting 4000 light photons emerging from the crystal only eject a total of 400 or so electrons from the photocathodes of all the photomultipliers. Statistical fluctuation in such a small number produces the range of pulse heights seen in the photopeak (see Fig. 5.5).

The pulse height analyzer – particularly in a sophisticated form called a multichannel analyzer – can be used to plot the photopeak (see Fig. 5.5). Its width, halfway up (FWHM), is defined as the energy resolution, and is typically 12% of the peak energy.

Setting a narrower pulse height analyzer window improves the energy resolution but reduces the sensitivity and increases imaging time. The energy resolution is better for high-energy gamma photons because they each produce more light photons. It is therefore better with ^{99m}Tc than with ^{201}Tl.

Temporal resolution: dead time and lost counts

The flash of light produced by a gamma photon in the crystal has a decay time of 0.2 μs. About 95% of the light has been emitted in 1 μs, at which point the pulse is cut off electronically. For that period the counting circuit does not recognize other pulses, and is said to be 'dead'. Due to the stochastic nature of radioactive decay, counts arrive at irregular intervals, as shown in Fig. 5.4. If a second gamma photon enters the camera during the dead time (indicated by vertical dashed lines in the figure) the two flashes of light overlap, and they are treated as one. If the combined pulse is too large, it will be rejected by the pulse height analyzer.

Lost counts. At high count rates a significant proportion of the gamma photons may be missed, and the count rate is underestimated. Typically there might be a 20% loss at 40 000 cps and more at higher count rates.

Effect on resolution. If two Compton-scattered photons (of say 60 and 80 keV) enter the system within 1 μs of each other they will be recorded as a single photon (140 keV, and able to pass through the pulse height analyzer) and produce a spurious image in a false location. At the high count rates in cardiac imaging this may cause deterioration of the spatial resolution.

Sensitivity

This is measured with a smaller version of the flood field phantom, and expressed as total counts per second per megabequerel of activity. Since the crystal efficiency is rather high, it is the collimator which determines overall efficiency. Up to a point, using a thicker crystal increases sensitivity at the expense of poorer resolution; more importantly, so does using a collimator with larger holes.

Noise: quantum mottle

Using a shorter exposure, the flood field phantom shows a characteristic mottled appearance. This is because the counts fluctuate from pixel to pixel. The computer can be instructed to draw a histogram of counts per pixel and to calculate the mean and standard deviation. Dividing the mean by the standard deviation gives the signal-to-noise ratio. Noise in gamma imaging is high because of the inherently small signal from a limited amount of radioactivity.

Noise could be reduced by using more radionuclide. However, the amount of radioactivity that may be administered to a patient is limited by the radiation dose to which the patient may be committed.

The activity is distributed through the body and typically only some 20% is concentrated in the organ of interest.

The gamma rays are emitted isotopically, and only a small fraction pass through the collimator holes, which cannot be made too large if resolution is not to be lost.

The gamma rays could be collected for any length of time without further dose to the patient, but the imaging time is limited by the ability of the patient to stay still and the workload required of the camera. The imaging time must be shorter still for dynamic studies, especially cardiac imaging.

The total counts acquired per image are further subdivided among the 128×128 pixels. This results in only about 100 counts per pixel, and so a pixel to pixel noise of 10%.

More important is the number of counts acquired over the blur size R – about 1000, with a noise of 3%. This allows hot spots and cold spots of about 10% to be detected against the background activity in the body. This 'contrast resolution' can only be improved at the expense of either increased patient dose or worsened spatial resolution.

Noise is the principal factor in determining the quality of gamma images. Gamma imaging is therefore said to be *noise limited* or dose limited. The count rate is maximized and the patient dose minimized by a judicious choice of radiopharmaceutical.

5.5 RADIOPHARMACEUTICALS

Desirable properties

Desirable properties of a *radionuclide* for imaging are:

◆ A physical half-life of a few hours, similar to the time from preparation to injection. If the half-life is too short, much more activity must be prepared than is actually injected.

◆ Decay to a stable daughter or at least one with a very long half-life (e.g. ^{99}Tc has half-life of 200 000 years).

◆ Emit gamma rays (which produce the image) but no alpha or beta particles or very low-energy photons (which have a high linear energy transfer, and only deposit dose in patient). Decay by isomeric transition or electron capture is therefore preferred.

◆ Emit gamma rays of energy 50–300 keV and ideally about 150 keV – high enough to exit the patient but low enough to be easily collimated and easily measured, being largely absorbed in the collimator septa and the crystal.

◆ Ideally emit monoenergetic gamma rays so that scatter can be eliminated by energy discrimination with the pulse height analyzer.

◆ Be easily and firmly attached to the pharmaceutical at room temperature but not affect its metabolism.

◆ Be readily available on the hospital site.

◆ Have a high specific activity.

In addition, the *radiopharmaceutical* should:

◆ localize largely and quickly in the 'target' – the tissues of diagnostic interest;

◆ be eliminated from the body with an effective half-life similar to the duration of the examination, to reduce the subsequent dose to the patient;

◆ have a low toxicity;

◆ form a stable product both *in vitro* and *in vivo*;

◆ be readily available and cheap per patient dose.

The decay during transport and storage of a short-lived radionuclide is reduced if it can be supplied with its longer-lived parent in a generator.

Technetium generator

^{99m}Tc is used in 90% of radionuclide imaging as it fulfills most of the above criteria. With its gamma energy of 140 keV, it is easily collimated and easily absorbed in a fairly thin crystal, thus giving good spatial resolution. With its short half-life and pure gamma emission, a reasonably large activity can be administered, reducing noise. It is supplied in a generator shielded with lead. As the simplified cross-section in Fig. 5.9 shows, this contains an alumina exchange column on which has been absorbed a compound of the parent ^{99}Mo (which can be produced in a reactor and has a 67 h half-life).

At the time of arrival, the activity of the 'daughter' ^{99m}Tc has built up to its maximum, equal to that of the parent ^{99}Mo. The daughter is decaying as quickly as it is being formed by the decay of its parent. It is said to be in transient equilibrium with the parent. The daughter and parent decay together with the half-life of the parent, 67 h (Fig. 5.10).

The technetium is washed off (*eluted*) as sodium pertechnetate with sterile saline solution. This flows under pressure from a reservoir through the column into a rubber-capped sterile container. The precise design of the

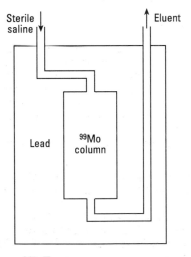

Fig. 5.9 Schematic diagram of ^{99m}Tc generator.

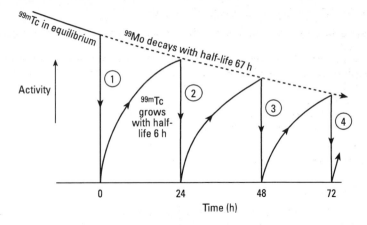

Fig. 5.10 Decay of activity of ^{99m}Mo and growth and regrowth of activity of ^{99m}Tc in a generator which is eluted daily.

generator and pressure system depends on the manufacturer. Elution takes a few minutes, and leaves behind the molybdenum, which is more firmly attached to the column.

Thereafter the eluent decays with its own half-life of 6 h. At the same time, the ^{99m}Tc in the column regrows with the same half-life of 6 h. After 24 h the activity has grown again to a new maximum (equilibrium) value. (After 6 h it has reached 50% of the maximum; after 12 h, 75% and so on.)

Figure 5.10 plots the activity of ^{99}Mo (dashed line) and ^{99m}Tc (solid line) against time, following the first elution (1) at time 0. Elution can be made daily – though it will be seen that the strength of successive eluents (2, 3, . . .) diminishes in line with the decay of ^{99}Mo. After a week, the generator is replaced and the old one is returned for recycling. If necessary, the column can be eluted twice daily.

Uses of technetium-99m

Sodium pertechnetate-99m is used for imaging the tissues which take it up, on account of its similarity to iodide and chloride ions: the thyroid (by which it is trapped but not fully metabolized), gastric mucosa (localization of Meckel's diverticulum), and the salivary glands. Blocked from the thyroid by administration of potassium perchlorate, it has been used for cerebral blood flow and testicular imaging, and, mixed with bran porridge, for gastric emptying studies.

Technetium can easily be labelled to a wide variety of useful compounds, for example:

- hexamethyl propylene amine oxime (HMPAO), for cerebral imaging;
- dimercaptosuccinic acid (DMSA) and mercaptoacetyltriglycine (MAG3) for renal studies;
- iminodiacetic acid (HIDA) for biliary studies;
- human serum albumin (HSA) colloidal particles, 0.5 μm in size, which are phagocytosed in reticulo-endothelial cells – imaging of liver, spleen and red bone marrow;

◈ HSA macroaggregates – 15–100 μm microspheres which temporarily block a small fraction of the capillaries in lung perfusion imaging;
◈ diethylene triamine pentacetic acid (DTPA) aerosol (5 μm particles) in lung ventilation studies
◈ diphosphonates, for bone imaging, being taken up in sites of bone repair;
◈ autologous red cells, for cardiac function;
◈ heat-damaged autologous red cells, for imaging the spleen;
◈ sestambi or tetrofosmin, for cardiac perfusion imaging.

The need for some of the above investigations has been reduced by the availability of other imaging modalities such as ultrasound.

Other radionuclides and their uses

Iodine is avidly trapped and metabolized by the thyroid, which was the organ first imaged, and *iodine-131* (^{131}I) the first radionuclide used for imaging. It was cheap, highly reactive, and an excellent label. It is produced in a reactor and has a long shelf life (half-life 8 days), but emits beta rays as well as rather energetic (mainly 364 keV) gamma rays. It has therefore largely been replaced by iodine-123 (^{123}I), which is more expensive, is cyclotron produced, has a half-life of 13 h, and decays by electron capture, emitting 159 keV gamma rays. It is also more expensive than, but otherwise superior to, ^{125}I, with its long half-life (60 days) and low photon energy (around 30 keV). It may be labeled to hippuran for renal studies, being cleared by both glomerular filtration and tubular secretion.

Xenon-133 (^{133}Xe) is produced in a reactor, has a half-life of 5.2 days and emits beta rays and rather low-energy (81 keV) gamma rays. It is an inert gas, although somewhat soluble in blood and fat, and is used, with rebreathing, in lung ventilation imaging.

Krypton-81m (^{81m}Kr), another inert gas, is generator produced, has a half-life of 13 s, and emits 190 keV gamma rays. The generator is eluted with compressed air, the patient inhaling the air–^{81m}Kr mixture in pulmonary ventilation studies. The short life of the parent (^{81}Rb, 4.7 h) presents transport difficulties, and means it must be used the day it is delivered.

Gallium-67 (^{67}Ga) is cyclotron produced, has a half-life of 78 h, and decays by electron capture, emitting gamma rays of three main energies. Gallium citrate is used to detect tumors and abscesses as it binds to plasma proteins.

Indium-111 (^{111}In) is cyclotron produced, has a half-life of 67 h, and decays by electron capture, emitting 173 and 247 keV gamma rays. It is used to label white blood cells and platelets for locating abscesses and thromboses, respectively.

Indium-113m (^{133m}In) is sometimes used instead of ^{111}I, is generator produced, has a half-life of 100 min, and emits only gamma rays, but they have a high energy (390 keV).

Thallium-201 (^{201}Th) is cyclotron produced, has a half-life of 73 h, and decays by electron capture, emitting 80 keV X-rays. An analog of potassium, it is used as thallous chloride in myocardial perfusion imaging, where its half-life is well suited to repeated imaging over a few hours.

Preparation of radiopharmaceuticals

This usually involves the simple mixing or shaking at room temperature of the radionuclide (e.g. ^{99m}Tc as sodium pertechnetate) with the compound to be labeled (e.g. methylene diphosphonate, MDP) and other necessary chemicals. Shielded syringes are used to transfer the components between sterile vials. The manipulations are carried out under sterile conditions in a 'workstation': a glove box or a laminar downflow cabinet which admits the entry of hands, etc., through a certain of air flowing down across the open face of the cabinet.

The cabinet is located in a room which is under a positive pressure of filtered sterile air. All surfaces are impervious: continuous floors, gloss-painted walls, and formica-topped benches. Entry is via an air lock and changing room. Normal sterile procedures are followed. The pharmacy must meet the conditions of both the Medicines Act and the Ionising Radiations Regulations (see Section 6.6) in the UK, or the relevant regulations in other countries.

Quality control includes testing for:

- *radionuclide purity* – testing for contamination with ^{99}Mo, which would give an unnecessary dose to the patient, by measuring any gamma radiation after blocking off the gamma rays from ^{99m}Tc with 6 mm lead (see also Section 5.6);
- *radiochemical purity* – testing for free pertechnetate in a labeled compound by chromatography;
- *chemical purity* – spot colour test for alumina, which may have come from the column and would interfere with labeling;
- *sterility testing and pyrogen testing* – the results of which are available only retrospectively, after the main part of the eluent has been used;
- *response of the radionuclide calibrator* (see Section 5.6).

5.6 DOSE TO THE PATIENT

Dose to an organ

The absorbed dose delivered to an organ by the activity it has taken up increases in proportion to:

- the activity administered to the patient and the fraction taken up by the organ;
- the effective half-life of the activity in the organ;
- the energy (MeV) of beta and gamma radiation emitted in each disintegration;

It also depends on how much of that energy escapes from the organ and so does not contribute to the absorbed dose. All the energy of a beta ray is deposited inside the organ and none escapes. Some of the energy of a gamma ray is deposited in the organ and some leaves it, to an extent depending on the size of the organ and how energetic the gamma ray is.

The calculation is complicated and must also take account of the additional dose delivered to the organ by gamma rays coming from activity in surrounding tissues and organs.

PHYSICS FOR MEDICAL IMAGING

Effective dose to the body

Unlike imaging with X-rays, the dose delivered by a radionuclide examination is unaffected by the number of images taken, and it is not confined to the region of diagnostic interest. After an intravenous injection most tissues may receive some dose, but the target organ and the organs of excretion generally receive the highest doses.

The distribution of a dose is nonuniform and specific to the examination, but an average dose to the body as a whole can be calculated. This is termed the effective dose (ED), which is measured in sieverts (Sv), and explained in Section 6.3. It also takes account of the differing sensitivities of different organs and tissues to irradiation.

Typical activities and doses

Most investigations deliver an ED of 1 mSv or less, which is no greater than the variation, from place to place and individual to individual, in the annual dose of natural radiation. Some, such as bone or static brain imaging, deliver doses in the region of 5 mSv, equal to the annual dose limit allowed for members of the general public. A few examinations, such as tumor or abscess imaging with ^{67}Ga, deliver higher doses, and are only to be undertaken when other imaging modalities are inappropriate (Table 5.2).

In order to minimize patient dose, patients should drink a good deal of water and empty the bladder frequently to reduce the dose to the gonads and pelvic bone marrow.

The activity of each administration of radiopharmaceutical is kept within the limits set by the Administration of Radioactive Substances Advisory Committee (ARSAC) of the UK Department of Health, or the relevant limits in other countries (see Section 6.6), and checked and recorded before administration. The phial is placed in the 'well' of a large re-entrant ionization chamber – *the radionuclide* or *dose calibrator*. The ionization current produced by the gamma rays is proportional to the activity of the sample but also depends on the gamma energy and half-life of the radionuclide being assayed. The radionuclide is entered on the control panel and the activity in megabecquerels is displayed on a digital read-out. The accuracy of the radionuclide calibrator must be checked regularly using a reasonably long-lived source, such as ^{57}Co. The calibrator

Table 5.2 Typical activities and doses

Site	Agent	Activity (MBq)	Effective dose (mSv)
Bone	^{99m}Tc phosphonate	600	5
Lung ventilation	^{99m}Tc DTPA aerosol	80	0.6
	^{81m}Kr gas	6000	0.1
Lung perfusion	^{99m}Tc HA macroaggregates	100	1
Kidney	^{99m}Tc DTPA gluconate	80	1
	^{99m}Tc MAG3	100	1
Tumor	^{67}GaGa^{3+}	150	18

can also be used with a lead sleeve to check for the higher-energy gamma rays from molybdenum breakthrough.

5.7 PRECAUTIONS TO BE TAKEN IN THE HANDLING OF RADIONUCLIDES

When handling radionuclides, in addition to the hazard from external radiation there is also a potential hazard from internal radiation due to accidental ingestion or inhalation of the radionuclide or its entry through wounds. It is therefore important to avoid contamination of the environment, the workplace, and persons, and to control any spread of radioactive materials. Generally, the risk from contamination is greater than that from external radiation.

Segregation

A nuclear medicine facility must have separate areas for (a) the preparation and storage of radioactive materials, (b) the injection of patients, (c) patients to wait, (d) imaging, and (e) temporary storage of radioactive waste. Patients containing radioactivity are a source of external radiation. They should be spaced apart in the waiting area. Departmental layout should make use of the inverse square law to reduce the effect of background radiation from other patients and sources, particularly in the imaging areas.

Personal protection

Use should be made of distance, shielding, and time. Staff should only enter areas where there is radioactivity when it is strictly necessary; all procedures must be carried out expeditiously and efficiently. Departmental local rules must be followed. Some general guidance follows.

Radionuclides are contained in shielded generators or in bottles in lead pots. Where feasible, bottles and syringes are handled with long-handled forceps (tongs). Manipulations, such as the labeling of pharmaceuticals and the loading of syringes, are carried out with the arms behind a lead barrier which protects the body and face, and over a tray, lined with absorbent paper, to catch any drips.

Syringes are protected by heavy metal or lead glass sleeves (which can reduce radiation doses by 75%) and are transported in special containers or on a kidney dish. Before injection, syringes are vented into swabs or closed containers and not into the atmosphere.

Lead–rubber aprons are ineffective against the high-energy gamma rays of ^{99m}Tc. To avoid accidental ingestion, waterproof (double-latex) surgical gloves are worn when handing radionuclides. Cuts and abrasions must be covered first. There must be no eating, drinking, or facial contact. Hands and work surfaces are routinely monitored for radioactive contamination, and the air in radiopharmacies may also be sampled and monitored. Staff will be monitored for external radiation doses to the body and possibly the hands. They may also be monitored for internal contamination. Swabs are taken from the workstation to monitor for radioactive and bacterial contamination.

Hands should be washed regularly at special wash basins. Where necessary, and particularly after spills, decontamination may be carried out. This normally involves the use of water, mild detergents, and swabs, which are then sealed in plastic bags and disposed of as radioactive waste in marked bins. Any use of a nail brush should be gentle; if contamination is obstinate, special detergent solutions may be necessary.

Patient protection

Every radionuclide should be checked for activity before administration, using a radionuclide ('well') calibrator. The patient's identity must be checked against the investigation to be made and the activity to be administered, and this must be recorded. Particular care should be taken to avoid contamination during oral administrations. Special circumstances apply for pregnant patients and those with babies they are breast-feeding.

Dealing with a radioactive spill

In the case of a radioactive spill, vomiting, incontinence, etc., clear the area of nonessential persons. Wearing gloves, aprons, and overshoes, mop the floor with absorbent pads and seal the swabs in designated plastic bags. If necessary, continue with wet swabs. Continue until monitoring shows the activity to be at a satisfactorily low level. If necessary, cordon off the area or cover it with impervious sheeting until sufficient decay has occurred. Contaminated materials are treated as waste.

Disposal of radioactive waste

These follow the two principles of:

◆ containment and decay; and
◆ dilution by dispersal to the environment.

Special rules and authorizations cover the accumulation, storage, and disposal of radioactive waste. Every hospital is subject to strict limitations on the amount which can be disposed of by each of the following routes.

Gaseous waste can be vented to the atmosphere: in lung ventilation studies, ^{133}Xe and ^{99m}Tc aerosols should be exhausted to the exterior of the building; this is not necessary with the very short-lived ^{81m}Kr.

Aqueous liquid waste may be disposed of, well diluted with water, via designated sinks or sluices with drains running direct to the foul drain.

Solid waste (swabs, syringes, bottles, etc.) are to be placed in designated sacks for disposal by incineration or, if suitably diluted with ordinary waste, to waste disposal sites. Old generators are kept in a secure shielded store until they are returned to the manufacturer.

Contaminated clothing and bedding is appropriately bagged and stored in a secure protected area until sufficiently decayed for release to the laundry.

Records must be kept, for inspection, of all deliveries, stocks, administration, stored waste, and disposals of waste.

5.8 TOMOGRAPHY WITH RADIONUCLIDES

Conventional 'planar' gamma imaging, so far described, produces a two-dimensional projection of a three-dimensional distribution of a radiopharmaceutical; the images of organs are superimposed, depth information is lost, and contrast is reduced. These deficiencies are overcome in emission tomography (ET), which uses the same principles as X-ray or transmission CT to reconstruct the images of a series of parallel body sections. There are two methods: *single-photon emission CT* (SPECT) and *positron emission tomography* (PET).

5.8.1 Single-photon emission computed tomography (SPECT or SPET)

A gamma camera with a parallel hole collimator rotates slowly in a circular orbit around the patient lying on a narrow cantilever couch. Every 6°, the camera halts for 20–30 s and acquires a view of the patient; 60 views are taken from different directions, each, however, comprising fewer counts than in conventional static imaging. Some 3 million counts are acquired in an overall scanning time of 30 min.

Figure 5.11 shows just two positions of the camera, which is represented schematically by its equivalent 64 × 64 pixel matrix. Each column, 64 pixels long and two or three pixels wide, like the one identified in the diagram, corresponds to a transverse slice through the patient. Each pixel corresponds to a line of sight, along which the counts or activity are summed – the emission analog of the fan beam in X-ray CT.

The 60 sets of data are synthesized, with some difficulty, into a transverse image by methods similar to those used in X-ray CT – *filtered back-projection*. This mathematical 'filtering' process can perhaps be understood more easily here than in the X-ray case. Referring to Fig. 4.14, within the computer memory frame, *negative* counts are projected along either side of the 'stripes' of true positive counts. A sufficient number of such stripes or projections add up to form a sharp image, free of star artefacts.

Thus, a stack of 20–30 transverse sections can be imaged simultaneously. If required, sagittal, coronal and oblique sections can be derived from them.

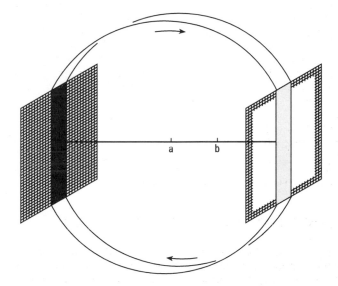

Fig. 5.11 Schematic arrangement of a SPECT imaging system.

It is also possible to display a continuously rotating three-dimensional representation exhibiting, among other things, surface texture of organs.

The considerable amount of *attenuation* that takes place in the patient would result in an image darker in the center than toward the edges. Allowance for this is made, by means of an algorithm, in reconstructing the image. This is made more precise by adding the counts, pixel by pixel, in each pair of opposing views (Fig. 5.11). The combined counts are then more nearly the same, whether the same amount of activity is near the center (a in Fig. 5.11) or near the edge of the patient's section (b).

SPECT images are severely photon limited *Noise* is high due to the limited number of counts in each voxel. Very few of the photons emitted in the patient are collected by the collimator holes corresponding to each slice. The overall imaging time is limited by patient movement, and photons are collected for only 20–30 s for each image. Noise could be reduced by making the slices thicker, but that would increase partial volume artefacts. The need to reduce noise limits the pixel matrix to 64×64 and the number of views to 60, i.e. 30 pairs. Noise can also be reduced by mathematical filtering, but at the cost of reduced spatial resolution.

Each slice is therefore reconstructed from only 64 measurements in each of 30 angular positions. On account of this and the need to use high-sensitivity collimators, the *spatial resolution* may be no better than 18 mm, i.e. about $3 \times$ pixel size. This is worse than a conventional gamma image and much worse than X-ray CT.

The image reconstruction process magnifies the effect of noise and also of any nonuniformity in the field. Automatic balancing of the photomultipliers is desirable. The photomultipliers would be affected by changes in their orientation, as the camera rotates, if they were not shielded from the earth's magnetic field. For similar reasons the gantry should be extremely well made. Maintenance and quality assurance are particularly important.

The camera must move on a sufficiently large circular orbit to miss the patient's shoulders. An elliptical orbit is sometimes used to minimize the gap between the collimator and the patient, and so improve resolution. Rotation of 180° is a useful option, e.g. in cardiac tomography. Some dedicated equipment uses two, three, or four gamma cameras equally spaced around the ring, thus increasing both speed and resolution.

As indicated above, SPECT studies can be presented either as a series of slices or as a *three-dimensional display*. The latter is particularly effective when the image is rotated continuously on the computer screen, showing defects in the organ. Thallium studies of myocardial infarctions and ischemia are major uses of SPECT, along with quantitative cerebral blood flow. Other applications, such as the detection of tumors and bone irregularities, are increasing in clinical usefulness as the algorithms which correct for tissue attenuation are improved.

5.8.2 Positron emission tomography (PET)

Positive beta emitters (e.g. ^{11}C, ^{13}N, and ^{15}O, isotopes of basic biological elements) prepared in the cyclotron and used as oxygen or carbon dioxide gas are employed in regional blood flow imaging. Unfortunately they have short half-lives (20, 10, and 2 min, respectively), and their use depends on a nearby cyclotron and radiochemical laboratory. Minicyclotrons have been designed specially for their production on site.

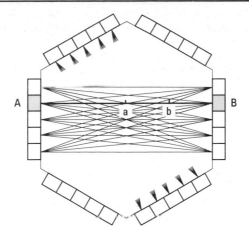

Fig. 5.12 Schematic arrangement of a PET imaging system.

After traveling for less than 1 mm through the patient, the positive beta particles is annihilated by a negative electron, whereupon two photons, each of exactly 511 keV, are emitted simultaneously and in practically opposite directions (but not exactly so, if the positron is moving when annihilated).

A *positron camera* comprises a ring, hexagon, or other polygon surrounding the patient and composed of a large number (e.g. 90 or 180) of photomultiplier tubes coupled to bismuth germinate detectors. If, as in Fig. 5.12, the annihilation photons enter detectors A and B, respectively, they produce simultaneous (coincident) pulses which are accepted and combined by the electronics. Any pulses which do not coincide in time are ignored by the electronics. These two detectors therefore measure only the sum of the activity present along a line AB – and similarly for each of the many pairs of detectors – which is just the information required for tomographic reconstruction, as in CT or SPECT.

Each detector can operate in coincidence with each of the facing 11 (or so) detectors, so that the patient is criss-crossed by hundreds of scan lines, some of which are shown in the diagram. The gaps between them can be reduced by a slight translation of the detectors and rotating the ring in twelve 5° steps during imaging. Single photons of background radiation entering only one detector are ignored and not counted.

The reconstruction algorithm includes a correction for *tissue attenuation*, but this is small and easily applied because of the high photon energy and because the combined distance travelled in tissue by the two photons is the same whether the annihilation took place at, for example, a or b in Fig 5.12. Quantitative measurements can therefore be made.

Despite the high photon energy, the bismuth germinate detectors are many times more *sensitive* than a conventional gamma camera, particularly because little or no collimation is required, apart from simple slit collimation to define the 15 mm slice. Noise is correspondingly low. The effective dose to the patient is much the same as in routine gamma imaging as the short life compensates for the beta emission.

Spatial resolution is impaired by random or accidental coincidences between the arrival of pairs of unrelated photons at the counters – caused, for example, by Compton scatter of the annihilation photons in the body. Overall resolution depends on the width or 'acceptance angle' of the detectors, and can be 5 mm or less, which is better than SPECT. It is the same at all depths, whereas in SPECT it worsens with increasing depth.

Other positron emitters which have been used in PET imaging include ^{18}F (half-life 112 min, used to label deoxyglucose, FDG), ^{68}Ga (68 min), and ^{82}Rb (1 min). The last two are produced by generators. PET imaging has stimulated the production of pharmaceuticals labeled with ^{123}I and ^{99m}Tc, able to cross the blood–brain barrier, for use in SPECT which has become a simpler and cheaper alternative to PET in cerebral blood flow imaging.

VIVA QUESTIONS

1 Why is technetium-99m so useful a radionuclide in gamma imaging?

2. How is technetium-99m generated?

3. Explain the construction and function of a gamma camera.

4. What properties are necessary for (a) a radionuclide and (b) a radiopharmaceutical to be successful in gamma imaging?

5. Explain the terms (a) physical half-life, (b) biological half-life, and (c) effective half-life of a radionuclide.

6. Draw the radionuclide decay of molybdenum-99 with the emissions produced.

7. Define a becquerel. What amounts are used in gamma imaging? Give some examples.

8. What is meant by 'exponential decay'?

9. What medically useful radionuclides are produced in a cyclotron?

10. What is the purpose of a collimator?

11. What types of collimator are there?

12. How does a gamma camera work?

13. How can you assure the quality of the gamma camera image?

14. What is (a) a pulse height analyzer and (b) a pulse height spectrum?

15. What is the difference between static and dynamic gamma imaging?

16. Why are gamma rays of between 100 and 200 keV the most suitable for imaging with a gamma camera?

17. Name some radionuclides (other than technetium-99m) that are used in imaging, with their energies and decay schemes.

18. What is SPECT, and why is it useful?

19. What is PET, and why is it useful?

20. What artefacts arise from a cracked crystal in a gamma camera?

21. Explain the use of photomultiplier tubes in a gamma camera.

22. In what types of radionuclide imaging are the following used: (a) iodine-123, (b) xenon-133, (c) thallium-201, and (d) gallium-67? What are their decay processes?

23. Name some chemical agents that can be labeled with technetium-99m, and state their use in imaging.

24. On what parameters does the absorbed dose to the patient depend? Give some examples of effective dose values for various radionuclide images.

25. What precautions for personal and patient protection are necessary during radionuclide administrations?

6

RADIATION HAZARDS AND PROTECTION

6.1 IONIZING RADIATION INTERACTIONS WITH TISSUE

When ionizing radiations, such as X- and gamma rays, interact with living tissue, it is the absorption of radiation energy in the tissues which causes damage. If the radiation passed through the tissue without absorption, there would be no biological effects and no radiological image would be produced. Whenever radiation is absorbed, chemical changes are produced virtually immediately, and subsequent molecular damage follows in a short space of time (seconds to minutes). It is after this, during a much longer time span of hours to decades, that the biological damage becomes evident (Fig. 6.1).

There are many examples of *radiation-induced damage*: to the skin and hands suffered by the early radiologists: excess leukemias in patients treated with radiation for ankylosing spondilitis; and radiation accidents in various parts of the world. However, the current estimates of radiation risk for cancer induction have been mostly derived from the outcomes, since 1945, of those exposed to nuclear explosions, particularly the 90 000 survivors of the atomic bomb attacks on Hiroshima and Nagasaki.

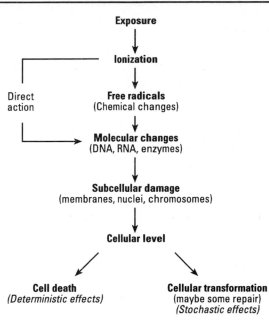

Fig. 6.1 Chain of events following exposure to ionizing radiation.

Medical radiation includes both particulate radiations (beta particles and neutrons) and ionizing electromagnetic radiations (gamma and X-rays). Although the principal radiation source for medical exposures is diagnostic X-rays, other important sources include gamma-emitting radionuclides in nuclear medicine and radiotherapy sources including beta emitters, electron beams, and gamma and X-ray sources.

Whenever a beta particle or an electron passes through tissue, ionizations and excitations occur repeatedly until eventually the particle comes to rest, giving up all of its energy. Being relatively light, such electrons are easily deflected by the negatively charged orbital electrons of the tissue atoms that they encounter, and so follow a very tortuous path. The total range involved in tissue interactions is of the order of a few millimeters at most. Hence electrons are relatively easily absorbed by a shield of several millimeters of Perpex or by thin sheets of metal, depending on their initial energy.

Unlike beta particles, X- and gamma radiations do not have a maximum depth of penetration associated with them but they simply undergo progressive attenuation. That is, the intensity of the radiation beam continues to fall as it interacts with tissue but at any given depth a residual beam always remains, however much less intense. (See also Chapter 1.)

During radiation exposures it is the *ionization* process that causes the majority of immediate chemical changes in tissue. The critical molecules for radiation damage are believed to be the proteins (such as enzymes) and nucleic acid (principally DNA). The damage occurs in two basic ways: by producing lesions in solute molecules directly, e.g. by rupturing a covalent bond, or by an indirect action between the solute molecules and the free radicals produced during the ionization of water.

Indirect damage arises more commonly because living tissue is about 70–90% water. If a pure water molecule is irradiated, it emits a free electron and produces a positively charged water ion, which immediately decomposes:

$$H_2O + \text{radiation} \rightarrow H_2O^+ + e^-$$

$$H_2O^+ \text{ decomposes} \rightarrow H^+ + OH^{\bullet}$$

The hydroxyl free radical $OH^{\bullet}$ is a highly reactive and powerful oxidizing agent which produces chemical modifications in solute organic molecules. These interactions, which occur in microseconds or less after exposure, are one way in which a sequence of complex chemical events can be started, but the free radical species formed can lead to many biologically harmful products and can produce damaging chain reactions in tissue.

The exact mechanism of these complex events is incompletely understood, but biological damage following exposure to ionizing radiations has been well documented at a variety of levels. Figure 6.1 shows the chain of events. At a *molecular level*, macromolecules such as DNA, RNA, and enzymes are damaged; at the *subcellular level*, cell membranes, nuclei, chromosomes, etc., are affected; and at the *cellular level*, cell division can be inhibited, cell death brought about, or transformation to a malignant state induced. Cell repair can also occur, and is an important mechanism when there is sufficient time for recovery between irradiation events.

6.2 RADIATION QUANTITIES AND UNITS

The system of quantities and units used in radiation protection is set out in Fig. 6.2. For each radiological procedure, we can calculate the *absorbed dose* (in milligrays) given to each of the tissues or organs in the persons irradiated.

Equivalent dose

We then take account of the type of radiation used, to determine a radiation quantity called the equivalent dose for the tissue or organ irradiated. This dose quantity can then be used to compare, for example, the lung doses given by different techniques such as a chest X-ray and a nuclear medicine scan.

The equivalent dose is the absorbed dose multiplied by a *radiation weighting factor*, which is an indication of the effectiveness of the radiation type compared with that of electrons in inducing cancers at low doses and low dose rates. As the energy from X- and gamma rays is absorbed through the production of secondary electrons, it is believed that all three types of radiation have the same effectiveness. So in most medical applications the equivalent dose is numerically equal to the absorbed dose in tissue. The biologically damaging effects of heavy particles, such as neutrons or alpha particles, is 10–20 times greater than that of electrons as their energy is completely deposited in a much shorter range of tissue. Like absorbed dose, the units of equivalent dose are joules per kilogram, but are given the special name of sievert (1 Sv = 1 J kg^{-1}). Most diagnostic medical exposures are expressed in millisieverts (mSv).

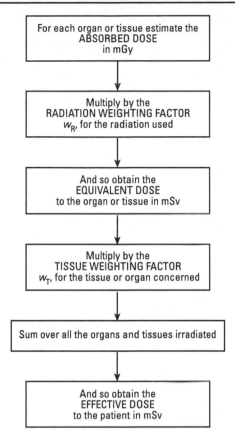

Fig. 6.2 Absorbed dose, equivalent dose, and effective dose.

The *effective dose* is the sum of the weighted equivalent doses for all the tissues which have been exposed, and is further explained at the end of Section 6.3. It also is expressed in sieverts. Occupational exposures are usually effective (whole-body) doses, and are expressed in microsieverts (μSv). If a person is uniformly irradiated by X- or gamma rays, the whole body absorbed dose, equivalent dose, and effective dose will have the same numerical values.

6.3 SOMATIC AND GENETIC EFFECTS OF IONIZING RADIATION

There are two categories of radiation effect: *somatic* effects which occur in the individual exposed and *genetic* or hereditary effects which occur in the descendants of those individuals as a result of lesions in the germinal cells.

Genetic effects

It is difficult to assess the genetic risk in humans, as even the descendants of those exposed at Hiroshima and Nagasaki have shown no additional genetic or cytogenetic effects. The frequency of congenital defects, fecundity, and life expectancy appear to be no different than for the children of nonirradiated parents. Similarly, surveys of descendants of radiotherapy patients show no increase in congenital defects. However, in view of the paucity of data, a safety margin is included in all risk estimates. The risk of hereditary ill-health in subsequent children or grandchildren is estimated to be at worst 10 extra cases from a million individual parents exposed to 1 mGy, whereas the normal incidence, without irradiation, is about 70 000 cases.

Deterministic effects

Somatic effects may be deterministic or stochastic (statistical). In the deterministic case a threshold dose applies, although it may be different for different persons. Once the threshold is exceeded, the severity of the effect increases with dose. Examples of deterministic (sometimes called nonstochastic) effects are cataracts, skin damage, bone marrow cell loss, and sterility. Biological damage cannot be identified at doses less than 50 mSv and in general, thresholds are greater than 500 mSv.

Damaging the lens of the eye is one of the highest deterministic risks. Cataracts are produced above a threshold of about 5 Sv to the lens. Computed tomography (CT) scans can give very high eye doses, and the possibility of damaging the eye lens in patients should not be forgotten. For skin damage the threshold for erythema and dry desquamation is about 4 Sv, and has been seen in some patients after interventional radiological procedures. Impairment of fertility varies with age, but 1 Sv to the gonads has a measurable effect and 4 Sv will cause sterilization.

The amount of radiation damage increases with the radiation dose, but it also increases with the volume of tissue irradiated and the rate at which the dose is given. For example, as the eye lens has no repair mechanism, the damage will be cumulative. If, however, the threshold dose for testicular damage is given in small amounts, say 1 mSv per week over a number of years, no deterministic effects will be observed.

Radiation doses which produce deterministic effects when only specific organs are irradiated will have a completely different effect if given as the same single absorbed dose, but this time to the whole body. For example, of a group of people exposed to 1.5 Sv whole body dose, half will show signs of radiation sickness (vomiting and diarrhoea) while the others may seem unaffected. Of a group exposed to 5 Sv, half will probably die within 30 days but half will recover if not exposed to infection. This value is known as the lethal dose (50% in 30 days) or $LD_{50/30}$. However, a whole body dose of 10 Sv or more is 100% lethal to humans, death being caused by a complete breakdown of the central nervous system, as well as the gastrointestinal tract.

Stochastic effects

In diagnostic radiology, where radiation doses are very small and deterministic effects should not occur, the somatic effects of real concern are the stochastic effects. For these, the probability of an effect occurring

Table 6.1 Organ-associated stochastic radiation risks

Organ	Mortality effect	Deaths per 1 mSv per million
Thyroid[a]	Cancer	0.8
Red bone marrow	Leukemia	5
Skin	Cancer	0.2
Bone	Cancer	0.5
Lung	Cancer	8.5
Breast[b]	Cancer	2
Esophagus	Cancer	3
Colon	Cancer	8.5
Liver	Cancer	1.5
Stomach	Cancer	11
Bladder	Cancer	3
Ovaries	Cancer	1
Remainder	Cancer	5
Total		*50*
Gonads[c]	Hereditary ill health	10

[a]Probability of induction is high but mortality is low.
[b]Age dependence ignored: breast is more sensitive during reproductive life.
[c]No hard evidence regarding hereditary effects: worse case prediction for one or two generations following irradiation.

(rather than its severity) increases with dose. This probabilistic effect is assumed to be a linear function of dose, with no threshold dose, for the induction of leukemias and solid tumors. Thus, cancer may be induced by very small doses of radiation.

Cancer induction actually has a latent period which ranges from a few years for leukemia up to perhaps 40 years for solid cancers. The radiation damage may therefore not be expressed within the lifetime of the recipient, depending on their age at exposure. Children are believed to be more radiosensitive than adults and, as they have a longer period in which to express any cancers, the risks associated with irradiating children are about three times those shown in Table 6.1. Irradiation *in utero* is considered to have special risks for the unborn child. Table 6.2 gives the best current estimates of risk, together with typical normal incidences in children. They are specially relevant to the radiological examination of women who are or might be pregnant (see Fig. 6.5) and the occupational exposure of female staff (see Section 6.5).

Probability coefficients for tissues at risk

The total risk of inducing a radiation detriment (fatal cancer, nonfatal cancer, or a hereditary effect) in a UK population of all ages and both sexes,

Table 6.2 Types of effect following irradiation *in utero*

Time after conception when irradiated	Effect	Deterministic threshold	Stochastic risk per 1 Gy	Normal incidence in live born infants
First 3 weeks	No deterministic or stochastic effects in live-born child			
Weeks 3–8	Potential for malformation of organs	100 mGy[a]		60×10^{-3} (1 in 17)
Weeks 8–25	Potential for severe mental retardation	120 mGy	4×10^{-3} (1 in 250)	5×10^{-3} (1 in 200)
Week 4 to term	Cancer in childhood or adult life		0.15×10^{-3} (1 in 7000)	1×10^{-3} (1 in 1000)

[a]Absorbed doses to the fetus as large as this are rarely encountered in diagnostic radiology, and recent re-analysis suggests that the threshold may even be 5–10 times higher.

which has been exposed to low doses at low dose rates of X-, gamma, or beta radiation to the whole body, is about 7% per sievert whole-body equivalent dose. This means that there is a likelihood of 7 in 100 of the effect occurring after an exposure of the whole group to 1 Sv. Assuming a linear relationship, it would also mean 70 cases in a million individuals each exposed to 1 mSv, which is a more realistic diagnostic equivalent dose. The risk can therefore be stated as *70 per million per 1 mSv*.

Each individual organ has an associated probability coefficient for fatal cancer induction, given in Table 6.1. These probability coefficients for organs are very approximate, containing a large number of uncertainties. Among the latter are uncertainties in the extrapolation from observed high dose, high-dose rate effects necessary to estimate the effects at low doses. (In the same group of 1 million there will also be 10 cases of nonfatal cancers, giving a total detriment of 70 cases.)

Effective dose

If the whole body has been exposed, then the total cancer mortality risk stated in Table 6.1 applies. If only part of the body has been exposed, for example during an X-ray procedure, the risk of dying from cancer relates to the risk only from the organs that have been exposed. To compare the risk from one procedure to that from another, an effective (whole-body) dose is calculated which gives the effective risk whether the whole body is irradiated uniformly or nonuniformly.

The effective dose is given by the sum of each organ dose multiplied by its relevant *organ weighting factor*. For example, an examination of the thoracic spine might give 1.3 mSv to the breast, 0.7 mSv to the red bone marrow, 2.8 mSv to the lungs, 1.5 mSv to the thyroid, and 1.5 mSv to bone. Using the organ or tissue weighting factors w_T in Table 6.3a would give an effective dose of about 0.6 mSv. The detailed calculation is given in Table 6.3b.

Note to Sections 6.2 and 6.3

In reading earlier literature, it may be helpful to know that, in 1990, radiation weighting factors replaced the radiation quality factors Q used

Table 6.3a ICRP[a] 60 (1991) tissue weighting factors

Tissue	w_T for each tissue	Σw_T
Gonads	0.20	0.20
Colon, lung, red bone marrow, stomach	0.12	0.48
Bladder, breast, liver, esophagus, thyroid	0.05	0.25
Bone, skin	0.01	0.02
Remainder — each of 5 organs/tissues	0.01	0.05
Total		1.00

[a]International Commission on Radiological Protection.

Table 6.3b Examination of the thoracic spine (example only)

Organs exposed	Equivalent dose to the organ (mSv)	Weighting factor, w_T	Weighted equivalent dose (mSv)
Breast	1.3	0.05	0.065
Red bone marrow	0.7	0.12	0.084
Lungs	2.8	0.12	0.336
Thyroid	1.5	0.05	0.075
Bone	1.5	0.01	0.015
Effective dose			0.575

previously and a new set of organ weighting factors was produced. This arose from the revision of the risk estimates for cancer induction determined from the Japanese radiation-exposed population. Prior to this date, the previous weighting factors dated back to 1977, when the quantity dose equivalent was used (now replaced by equivalent dose), and the effective dose equivalent was used to assess risk (now replaced by effective dose). The calculated values of effective dose are often lower than those of effective dose equivalent, but do not usually differ by more than 10% for a given diagnostic examination. However, the overall risk is thought to be 3–4 times higher than was thought to be the case 20 years ago.

6.4 IONIZING RADIATION CONTRIBUTIONS TO POPULATION EXPOSURE

Everyone is exposed to natural background radiation to a greater or lesser extent dependent on where they live and what they eat. Artificial or man-made sources of radiation also contribute to individual overall exposure. In the UK the annual *per caput* value for all radiation sources is about 2.6 mSv. Figure 6.3 shows the various contributions in pie chart form.

The largest contributor from natural background is exposure to radon gas, which permeates through the ground and into buildings. This averages about 1.3 mSv, but ranges widely from negligible to over 50 mSv, depending on the local geology. Gamma rays from the ground and building materials contribute about 350 μSv per year, and intakes of natural long-lived radionuclides in our food and drink contribute another 300 μSv. Cosmic radiation is reasonably constant at 260 μSv per year, although frequent air travelers could double their overall background dose as the cosmic ray dose rate increases considerably with altitude.

Out of the total 2.6 mSv *per caput* annual dose 2.2 mSv comes from natural radiation. Of the remaining 0.4 mSv from artificial sources, diagnostic medical radiation is the largest artificial source, at 0.37 mSv *per caput* annual dose. This means that we have a special responsibility to

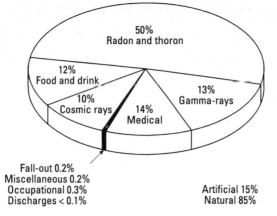

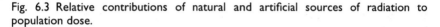

Fig. 6.3 Relative contributions of natural and artificial sources of radiation to population dose.

keep radiation exposures as low as possible when using diagnostic medical radiation.

6.5 RADIATION PROTECTION PRINCIPLES

The system of radiation protection proposed by the International Commission on Radiological Protection (ICRP) has long been incorporated into UK legislation. Although updated recently (1991) and likely to modify European and consequently UK legislation by the year 2000, the three fundamental principles remain. They are shown in outline in Fig. 6.4 and detailed below.

Justification

The benefit of the radiation exposure should be greater than the risk of using it whether this applies to staff, visitors or patients. Even though there are more *staff* using medical radiation than for any other use of radiation, they are not, in general exposed to such an extent as to offset the medical benefits either to the patient or to society.

When applied directly to the exposure of *patients*, the justification principle means that each particular medical practice in a department, for example chest X-ray to follow up pneumonia, must be justified both as a general procedure and then as regards the individual patient before the latter undergoes the procedure. Clearly, some exposures are easier to justify than others, while some are obviously unjustified. An example of the latter would be mammography screening in 20–30-year-old well-women, because it would probably cause more harm than benefit. Each department has procedures to follow for ensuring that patients are only subjected to justified procedures. When an individual patient falls outside the anticipated selection procedure, an individual justification must be made by the radiologist or nuclear medicine consultant. If the patient has been examined radiologically at another hospital recently for the same condition, every effort should be made to obtain the films and reports.

Sometimes an individual exposure is unjustified as the diagnosis can be made otherwise, for example using ultrasound, magnetic resonance imaging (MRI), or endoscopy, or would not actually contribute to the patient's management, for example in coccydynia.

Pregnant patients. A special case where individual justification is needed is for patients *who are or might be pregnant.* This follows the '28 day rule', outlined in Fig. 6.5. It applies to the radiographic examination of any area between the knees and the diaphragm and to the injection of radionuclides. It is based on the principle that there is little or no risk to the *live-born* child from irradiation during the first 3 weeks or so of gestation, i.e. before the first missed period; except possibly from high-dose procedures, such as barium enemas and abdominal or pelvic computed tomography (CT).

Figure 6.5 indicates the special care that must be taken when such examinations have to carried out on pregnant patients. In most cases, the dose equivalent to a fetus is unlikely to be as much as 5 mSv, and so the actual risk of inducing cancer in the child, taken from Table 6.2, is about 1 in 1000. This is about the same as the natural prevalence for malignancy before the 10th birthday.

Another special case is when radiopharmaceuticals are to be administered to a breast-feeding patient. If the radioactivity intake by the infant is likely to be high, breast-feeding may need to be interrupted or stopped.

Optimization

For members of staff or visitors the effective dose should be *as low as reasonably practicable* as constrained by the working procedures.

For a patient, the radiation exposure should be as low as compatible with providing the diagnostic information required. This can be achieved by *reducing the number of images* taken of a patient; for example the Royal College of Radiologists recommends only a posteroanterior chest view for chest trauma as oblique rib views do not alter management.

Another way to reduce the patient's dose is by *reducing the absorbed dose per image.* In this case, departmental policies need to be established with appropriate procedures to reduce patient dose, for example both with regard to dose-saving equipment and to the radiographic techniques used for individual examinations. Detailed guidance is given in Table 6.4. One of the best ways to optimize patient exposures in the department is to have a comprehensive *quality assurance* system which includes periodic measurements of patient doses. (See Sections 2.7.5, 3.3, 3.8, 3.10, 4.1.4, 4.2.4, 4.3.3, 5.4, 5.6, and 6.7.)

Limitation

There are legal dose limits for workers and members of the public, based on ensuring that no deterministic effects are produced and that the probability of stochastic effects is reasonably low. Limits are not appropriate for patients although 'reference values' have been published to indicate levels above which exposures should be reviewed (see Section 6.7). They include maximum values of activity for radiopharmaceutical administrations.

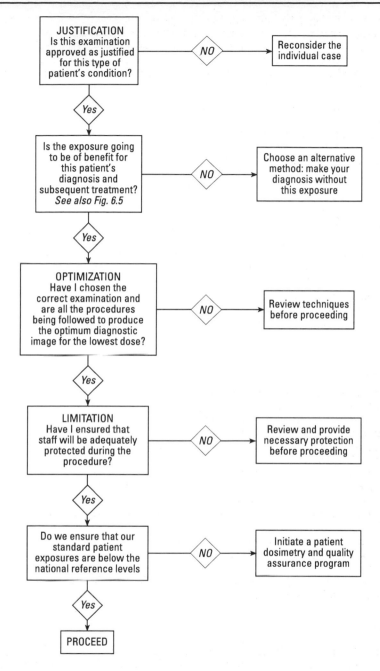

Fig. 6.4 Radiation protection principles applied to medical diagnostic procedures.

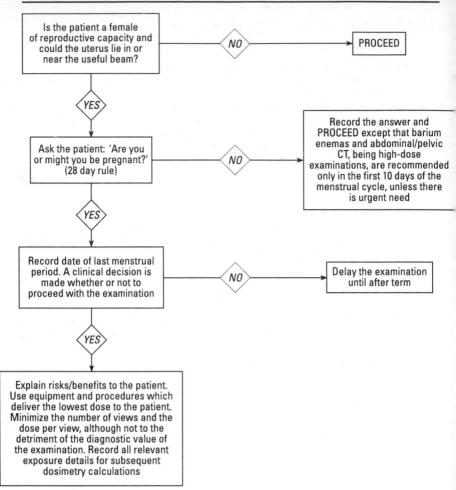

Fig. 6.5 Radiation protection of patients who are or might be pregnant.

The current dose limits (in UK law since 1985) are shown in Table 6.5. Staff who are likely to exceed 30% of any of the annual dose limits for workers need to be designated as 'classified', and their records kept centrally by the Health and Safety Executive (HSE). Such workers are *subject to regular medical surveillance* and must be monitored by dosimetry services which have been 'approved' by the HSE.

In practice, as shown in Fig. 6.6, staff working in radiodiagnostic imaging departments generally receive occupational doses less than 3 mSy per annum. Few are likely to exceed the current *public* dose limit. Even interventional radiologists, if they take appropriate care, should not exceed 30% of the annual occupational limits.

In view of the changes in risk estimates since 1990, dose limits are currently under review in the UK to see if they should be reduced to

Table 6.4 Practical measures for the reduction of patient dose

(a) *Some dose-saving equipment*

1. Fast screen–film combinations (e.g. rare earth)
2. Low attenuation (e.g. carbon fiber) materials for cassette fronts, antiscatter grid interspacing, table tops
3. Constant potential generators with appropriate kilovoltage
4. Appropriate beam filtration (minimum 2.5 mm Al for general radiography)
5. Specialized equipment for mammography and pediatrics
6. Pulsed and frame-hold (image storage) fluoroscopy equipment
7. Digital radiography equipment
8. Dose–area product meter to monitor patient exposure

(b) *Some dose-saving techniques*

1. Use smallest possible field size and good collimation
2. Collimate to exclude radiosensitive organs (gonads, breasts, eyes)
3. When gonads lie outside the primary beam, make distance between the edge of the field and the gonads as large as possible
4. Shield breasts, eyes, and gonads unless the area of interest would be masked. Dose to ovary can be halved and that to testes reduced by a factor of 20
5. Use largest practicable focus to skin distance: never less than 30 cm, especially in mobile radiography
6. Position the patient carefully. Reduce the dose to the female breast and, in skull radiography, to the eye by posteroanterior projection. Minimize the gap between patient and film–screen
7. Use compression of patient where possible
8. Use nongrid techniques when examining children and small adults
9. Keep film reject rate due to all causes down to 5%. Check the factors before exposure. Quality assurance, particularly of automatic processors, is important
10. In fluoroscopy use the minimal field size and minimal screening time essential for good diagnosis
11. Use zoom or small field techniques, which require a higher dose rate, with discretion

(c) *High-risk examinations*

1. Keep pediatric radiation doses to an absolute minimum consistent with adequate diagnosis as children up to the age of 10 years are believed to be 3–4 times more radiosensitive than adults
2. In pelvimetry: use MRI or CT scanography where possible; otherwise use fast rare earth screens and carbon fiber components
3. Mammography is not generally performed on women younger than 50 years unless there is a family history of breast cancer or the patient has related symptoms
4. In CT scanning, take the minimum number of slices, position the patient to avoid the eyes and other critical organs; reduce milliamperage if appropriate, e.g. for the chest
5. Patients who are or might be pregnant: see Fig. 6.5
6. Interventional radiology needs care to avoid skin reactions; use pulsed and frame-hold systems: minimize screening times

Table 6.5 Current UK dose limits (1985 Regulations)

	Dose limit (mSv)		
	Staff	Trainees aged 16–18 years	Public, visitors
Whole body	50	15	5
Eyes	150	45	15
Extremities and other organs	500	150	50

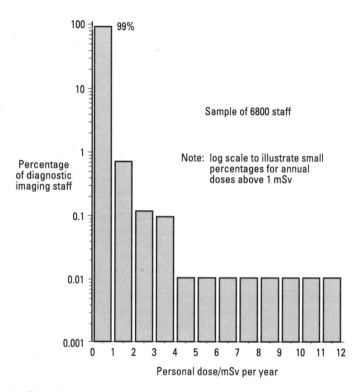

Fig. 6.6 Typical dose distributions among personnel in radiodiagnostic imaging departments.

maintain the same level of overall risk. Any new legal limits (which are not expected before 1998) are likely to reflect the changes in risk estimates relating to stochastic effects. Dose limits to the eyes and extremities are unlikely to change. The whole body annual dose limit may reduce to 20 mSv, and for the public may reduce to 1 mSv. In practice, the change may require more staff to be classified, for example if they are likely to exceed 6 mSv in a year.

All classified persons must wear personal dosemeters, and their dose and medical records are kept for 50 years after the last entry. Radiologists, and indeed nearly all radiation workers in hospitals, do not need to be designated as classified but are almost certainly required by the local rules to wear personal dosemeters when entering controlled areas.

Personal monitors are usually worn on the trunk, under any protective clothing. Additional monitors may be worn on the forehead or neckband if eye doses, or on the finger if hand doses, are likely to be significant. Body monitors are normally worn for 4 weeks, which is both sufficiently long for the accumulated dose to be large enough to be measured with sufficient accuracy, and sufficiently short for overexposures to be detected and their cause to be investigated reasonably quickly.

Personal monitors are usually either film badges or thermoluminescent dosemeters (TLD), the latter being particularly convenient as finger dosemeters. Electronic dosemeters can also be used in high-dose areas when an indication is needed at the time of the dose accrued, for example during interventional procedures by a pregnant radiologist. See Section 6.9 for details of the different systems.

Occupational exposure of fertile women

There are special limits to ensure that a fetus is not unduly exposed because of the occupational radiation exposure of the mother. Female staff should not be exposed to spasmodic high doses and on average should not receive more than about 1 mSv a month. There should be no need for any member of staff working in medical radiodiagnosis to exceed this particular figure.

Occupational exposure during pregnancy

Once a pregnancy has been declared, the occupationally exposed mother should not receive more than 10 mSv, averaged over her abdomen, for the remainder of pregnancy. In diagnostic radiology this would mean a maximum dose to the fetus of about 6 mSv. The future new limits are likely to lower the 10 mSv current dose limit to 2 mSv, thereby reducing the maximum effective fetal dose to about 1.2 mSv. Very few staff exceed these limits even now (Fig. 6.6).

6.6 STATUTORY RESPONSIBILITIES AND ORGANIZATIONAL ARRANGEMENTS FOR RADIATION PROTECTION

Key UK legislation

The requirements for the safe use of ionizing radiations in health care in the UK are defined for staff and members of the public by the *Ionising Radiations Regulations 1985 and the Ionising Radiations Regulations (Northern Ireland) 1985* (IRR 85) together with the *Radioactive Substances Act 1993*. For patients they are defined by the *Ionising Radiation (Protection of Persons Undergoing Medical Examination or Treatment) Regulations 1988 and the Ionising Radiation (Protection of Patients) Regulations (Northern Ireland) 1988* (IRR[POPUMET] 88) and also by *The Medicines (Administration of Radioactive Substances) Regulations 1978* (M[ARS]R 78).

All of this legislation is supplemented by Approved Codes of Practice and by Guidance Notes (see Bibliography), the latter of which give detailed practical recommendations on how the legislation should be implemented locally in the X-ray and nuclear medicine departments.

6.6.1 Protection of staff and members of the public

The legislation is enacted to ensure that individual doses are as low as reasonably practicable. This is achieved by ensuring premises and practices are designed so that people are most unlikely to exceed a proportion of the set dose limits.

Controlled areas

Protection begins at the source of the radiation, i.e. the X-ray tube or the syringe of radiopharmaceutical, and requires shielding to reduce the radiation exposure from the source. Where this cannot be reduced to a reasonable level, i.e. where constant exposure to the shielded source would mean that even 3/10 of dose limits (e.g. 15 mSv whole-body dose) were exceeded, a further control is introduced. The area around the source is designated as a *controlled area*, and this has to have defined physical boundaries which should prevent the penetration of the radiation above specified levels.

Every diagnostic X-ray tube produces a large amount of radiation exposure, and so by definition has to be contained within a controlled area (Fig. 6.7). This is simple to achieve in an X-ray room where the walls can be designed to protect to the necessary level of public exposure, but is more

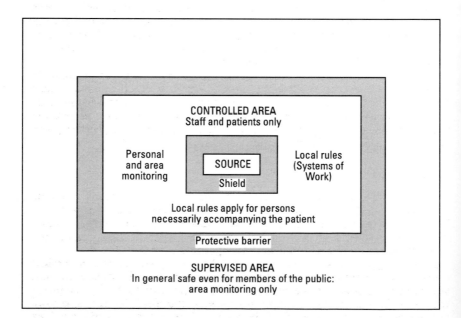

Fig 6.7 Controlled and supervised areas.

difficult with a mobile X-ray set. For the latter, a radiographer will determine the 'controlled area' by eye as extending for 2 m around the tube and patient while the X-ray is being taken. In nuclear medicine an area is defined as controlled wherever a generator is located or there is a syringe containing a radiopharmaceutical for injection. Section 5.7 details various protection requirements.

A controlled area has to be clearly defined and is controlled through restricting access to those staff who have been classified as radiation workers or to others who may work in that area but only under a 'written system of work'. The latter ensures that they cannot receive doses in excess of 3/10 of any dose limit. For example, staff working with X-ray equipment should be protected, either with screens (lead equivalence 2.5 mm) or with a lead–rubber apron, gloves, and lead glass spectacles (each of 0.2–0.5 mm Pb equivalence) as appropriate.

In practice, almost all diagnostic radiology and nuclear medicine staff receive doses which are below the public dose limit. They work in controlled areas under written systems of work (incorporated into the department's Local Rules), and there is no need for them to be classified.

Local Rules

Local Rules specify the procedures needed to ensure compliance with the Regulations. They include paragraphs on the safety organization, descriptions of the controlled areas, and the systems of work for working in the controlled areas and for restricting access to them. They also include the contingency plan for the department, in the event of a radiation incident. The system of work will include the need for lead protection if staff are working near the patient being radiographed but take account that, for example, distance and short contact time are more useful protectors in nuclear medicine when injecting and positioning patients. Staff will be monitored, and careful scrutiny of doses and feedback of dose information helps clinicians and others to decide the best way to undertake the various radiological procedures so as to keep staff doses as low as possible.

Local Rules are a legal document, and ignoring them is tantamount to breaking the law. Anyone finding their Local Rules to be impracticable should discuss them and get them changed by agreement so that compliance is easier. The Local Rules are 'policed' by a locally appointed radiation protection supervisor (RPS), often a senior radiographer, and enforced by the local HSE inspector.

Classified and other workers

If, for some reason, it is decided that a medical radiation worker should be a classified worker, an appointed doctor then takes an overview of the radiological health of the particular worker. Health and radiation monitoring become statutory, and all radiation dose records are submitted to a Central Index of Dose Information, operated for the HSE.

Recent legislation relating to classified working within the controlled areas of employers other than their own (for example when working on a seconded or consultancy basis for another employing authority) requires the individual to be issued with a *radiation passbook* by the approved dosimetry service to enable them to work within any controlled area. The passbook should contain their personal details and up-to-date radiation

Table 6.6 Differences between classified and other staff working in controlled areas

	Classified	Not classified
Annual effective dose limit	50 mSv	15 mSv
Personal monitoring	Required	Preferable
Follow 'system of work'	Preferable	Required
Medical surveillance	Required	Not required
Radiation passbook	Required for 'outside' work	

doses before entry to the controlled area is allowed. The dose received during work within the controlled area is then entered in the passbook when the individual leaves the area.

Having said that, most medical workers will not need to be classified but will be working under written systems of work to enter controlled areas (Table 6.6). Patients, of course, are present in the X-ray room, but only for their radiological examinations. The question of patients' relatives and other visitors to the X-ray department, such as X-ray engineers, is more difficult, and has to be covered by specific written systems of work in the Local Rules.

Legal liability (IRR 85)

All employers using ionizing radiation in controlled areas in which staff work are required by law to appoint a radiation protection adviser (RPA) to provide advice on the practical means of complying with legislation. All new work with ionizing radiation should be notified to the HSE 28 days before starting or significantly changing the work.

Anyone using ionizing radiation in a self-employed capacity with their own equipment is defined as the 'employer', and personally carries responsibility for all of the regulations, starting with notification to the HSE.

Most of the legislation lays 'duty of care' on the employer, so that the employer is responsible for ensuring the regulations are followed. A radiation protection committee is often used for this task. However, each employee has a duty to protect himself or herself, to ensure that they do not irradiate others inappropriately and to notify the employer of any suspected radiation incidents. Individuals should also follow the Local Rules, which are the local interpretation of the legislation, produced by or on behalf of the employer. It is obviously important that the employer should know of any deficiencies in compliance, and each department will have a system in place to ensure that this happens and that individuals understand the legal requirement to report problems. Employers have the responsibility for providing adequate training under IRR 85 and for ensuring prior training for staff clinically and physically directing exposures under IRR [POPUMET] 88 as described below.

The HSE has the responsibility of enforcing the *Ionising Radiations Regulations 1985*, and has the power to prosecute the employer or the individual worker under civil or criminal law. The 'employer' will be the person at the top of the organizational tree which has an employment contract with the worker concerned, e.g. the chief executive of a hospital. Liability may, however, be shared with other individuals through civil actions initiated by the 'employer' or through normal employment disciplinary procedures (Table 6.7).

Radioactive substances (RSA 93)

The acquisition, storage, and safe disposal of any radioactive substance is covered within the IRR 85 by the RSA 93. This Act controls radioactive substances in the environment, and so authorization for the accumulation and disposal of radioactive materials comes under the auspices of the Environment Departments. The requirements to comply with this Act are the responsibility of the employer, and are discussed further in Section 5.7.

6.6.2 Protection of patients

The IRR[POPUMET] 88 regulations are mainly concerned with the appropriate use of radiation procedures on patients, by staff who have been properly trained. The regulations outline the theoretical knowledge (called the 'core of knowledge', and set out in Table 6.8) that staff should have, and specify the need for practical instruction for all staff whether they are irradiating the patient directly, or carrying clinical responsibility for the patient's exposure. In the legislation, these latter two aspects are referred to, respectively, as 'physically' or 'clinically' directing the exposure. An individual not deemed to be fully trained may physically direct an exposure as part of their training only while under the supervision of a person who is adequately trained.

Regulation 4 of POPUMET is fundamental to patient protection and, in essence, requires every medical exposure to be carried out under the direction of a person who is *clinically directing* the exposure. This radiologist, for example, should ensure that only accepted diagnostic practices are used and that persons who are *physically directing* the exposure select procedures which ensure that the dose to the patient is as low as reasonably practicable, consistent with the requirements for diagnosis; these are the justification and optimization principles referred to in Section 6.5. Particular care should be taken over pregnant patients.

Referrals

A request from a general practitioner, for example, to a department for a radiological procedure, whether using X-rays or radionuclides, is interpreted as a request for an opinion. The importance of a properly filled in request form, as a legal document signed by a doctor, must be emphasized. The radiologist takes responsibility for clinical direction, and the radiographer for physical direction. This applies to procedures within the X-ray department and those outside on wards and in theaters where radiology department staff are directly involved. There are parallel responsibilities for nuclear medicine.

Referrals to radiology should be along clearly defined lines according to locally agreed referral criteria. The Royal College of Radiologists' handbook *Making the Best Use of the Radiology Department* is frequently used as a basis for local referral practice. (Documents of this sort are not legally binding; they represent good clinical practice but

Table 6.7 Legal liability and inspection

Area	Legislation			
	IRR 85	IRR[POPUMET] 88	M(ARS)R 78	RSA 93
Area	X-rays and nuclear medicine	X-rays and nuclear medicine	Nuclear medicine	Nuclear medicine
Liability	Employer and employee	Employer and practitioner	Employer and practitioner	Employer
Inspection	HSE	HSE and Government Health Departments	Departments of Health and of the Environment	Departments of the Environment

Table 6.8 Core of knowledge in the POPUMET regulations

1. Nature of ionizing radiation and its interaction with tissue
2. Genetic and somatic effects of ionizing radiation and how to assess their risks
3. The ranges of radiation dose that are given to a patient with a particular procedure, the principal factors which affect the dose and the methods of measuring such doses
4. The principles of quality assurance and quality control applied to both equipment and techniques
5. The principles of dose limitation and the various means of dose reduction to the patient including protection of the gonads
6. The specific requirements of women who are, or who may be, pregnant and also of children
7. If applicable, the precautions necessary for handling sealed and unsealed sources
8. The organizational arrangements for advice in radiation protection and how to deal with a suspected case of overexposure
9. Statutory responsibilities
10. In respect of the individual diagnostic and therapeutic procedures which the person intends to use, the clinical value of those procedures in relation to other available techniques used for the same or similar purposes
11. The importance of utilizing existing radiological information – films and/or reports – about a patient

have not yet been proven in law.) Locally specified procedures for the examination are then followed.

Other medical staff may personally take responsibility for clinical direction and/or physical direction, for procedures such as orthopedic surgery or cardiac catheterization using image intensifier fluoroscopy equipment. A doctor asking a radiographer to screen with such equipment is sharing responsibility for physical direction. Any radiographer who continues with a procedure knowing that it is inappropriate is equally culpable in law. This possible source of professional conflict should be managed with sensitivity.

Legal liability (IRR 88)

The legal obligations under the *Ionising Radiation (POPUMET) Regulations 88* are divided between those responsibilities which apply specifically to the employer and those which apply to the persons either clinically or physically directing procedures. In the latter case, responsibility for enforcement rests with the Secretary of State for Health, who uses the appropriate Health Department's Inspectorate (Table 6.7). There is in this case no 'umbrella' of an employer, and prosecutions or actions are directly against the individual responsible for particular procedures on particular patients. The employer may also wish to invoke normal employment disciplinary procedures.

Legal liability (M[ARS] regulations)

Diagnostic and therapeutic uses of radiopharmaceuticals are controlled by the M[ARS] Regulations of 1978 in addition to POPUMET. In practice, procedures should only be carried out under the clinical supervision of a person holding a certificate issued by the Administration of Radioactive Substances Advisory Committee (ARSAC) of the Department of Health. Administrations (physical direction) may be performed by other staff, specifically identified and instructed by the ARSAC Certificate holder for procedures authorized (both as to the pharmaceutical and the prescribed activity) in the ARSAC Certificate. The maximum does to the patient is defined in the Certificate by the maximum activity which may be administered.

ARSAC Certificates are issued to individual clinicians for specified procedures (including research) using specified equipment with scientific support. The application also has to be signed by the RPA. They are usually valid for up to 5 years (2 years for research). ARSAC Certificate holders and other persons physically directing the certificated procedure should also have been trained under IRR[POPUMET] 88. The employer is responsible for ensuring that the relevant clinicians hold current certificates. The clinicians are then responsible for the patients under M[ARS].

The responsibility for discharging radioactive patients from hospital lies with the ARSAC Certificate holder. Guidance is provided on the maximum activities remaining in the body which are deemed to be acceptable under defined circumstances for the patient to be discharged; and may require specific behavioral instructions or advice to the patient. The RPA should be able to advise further.

Equipment used for radiodiagnosis and treatment (IRR 85 Regulation 32)

Employers using medical X-ray equipment have to ensure that all such equipment is selected, installed, and maintained so that diagnosis and treatment can be carried out with minimum dose to the patient. This requirement extends to ancillary equipment which directly affects the dose to the patient, e.g. film processors, intensifying screens, radionuclide dose calibrators, etc. This is a statutory requirement under IRR(85) Regulation 32, and has been augmented through guidance from the HSE (PM77 1992). There is also guidance from the National Health Service (NHS) Management Executive on purchasing radiology equipment for patient dose-reduction (HSG[91]11).

Newly installed equipment should be subjected to a critical safety examination carried out by an RPA appointed by the installer, in addition to radiological acceptance testing and commissioning and subsequent periodic testing. Regular and frequent *quality assurance* should be carried out on those components which affect diagnostic quality and radiation dose. (Details can be found in the preceding chapters.) There should also be a log for the recording of faults and defects for each X-ray unit.

It is accepted that equipment *malfunctions* may occur from time to time. Consequently it is vital that systems are in place to detect and to correct for malfunctions and drift in performance. Deterioration in performance does not necessarily mean that equipment should be withdrawn from use.

However, it may mean that certain procedures should no longer be carried out using that equipment. Use of equipment which does not meet specifications for its original use should be properly justified (see Section 6.5) for any other uses.

Patient overexposures (IRR 85 Regulation 33)

The legislation has been designed to reduce the potential for errors in radiation administration to patients. However, human errors do occur and, when serious, will be investigated by the Department of Health. On the other hand, occasionally a patient may be overexposed because of an *equipment fault*. If the overexposure is greater than three times the dose that was intended (see Section 6.7), the following action is necessary:

- The manager responsible for the equipment (and the RPS) should be informed.
- The equipment should be withdrawn from use (in consultation with the RPA). The equipment should only be returned into use once the fault has been investigated and rectified.
- Details of the malfunction should be properly recorded, including the circumstances, equipment settings, patient details, who was present, etc.
- The dose received by the patient should be estimated by an RPA.
- The RPA will provide advice on further action as appropriate to the circumstances.

The Department of Health should always be informed of equipment failures so that hazard warning notices can be issued nationally as appropriate. The HSE should be informed in case of high-dose procedures (Table 6.9a), for compliance with IRR 85 Regulation 33.

As with all incidents, the hospital management should be informed, through the manager responsible for the equipment, once the details are clearly identified, and any established external reporting mechanisms should be followed.

Patient records

A record should made of the type of examination, radionuclide and activity administered, number of X-ray films and screening times, exposure factors and equipment used, film cassette size, and focus–skin distance, and the information kept for future reference, preferably in the patient's notes. This information may be needed for possible future litigation and is necessary for the calculation of 'total patient dose'. The Department of Health recommends that films and other records be kept for a minimum of 6 years. A properly completed request form, signed by a medical practitioner, is a legal document and should be retained, often in the patient's X-ray film packet.

6.7 PATIENT DOSIMETRY

Patient protection techniques have already been discussed in this chapter and in Chapter 5. The end point is to ensure that the patient receives no more dose than is necessary for the diagnosis. Measurements can be made using thermoluminescent (TL) chips (see Section 6.9.2) directly on the surface of a patient, or on a standard phantom. A dose–area product meter

Table 6.9a Ranges of effective dose

Effective dose	Range (mSv)	Procedure
High	5–50	Barium enema, gallium scan, CT scans
Medium	0.5–5	Intravenous urography, barium meal, lumbar spine, abdomen, pelvis, thoracic spine; ^{99m}Tc scans of brain, bone, kidney, liver, lung perfusion, thyroid imaging
Low	0.05–0.5	Chest, dental, skull

Table 6.9b Typical values of effective dose for a patient

	Procedure	Effective dose
Radiography	Chest X-ray	0.2 mSv
	Intravenous urography	5 mSv
	Barium meal	5 mSv
	Barium enema	9 mSv
	CT head scan	2 mSv
	CT abdomen scan	8 mSv
Fluoroscopy	Skin absorbed dose rate	20 mGy min^{-1}
	Effective dose rate	1 mSv min^{-1}
Gamma imaging	Abscess imaging (^{67}Ga: 150 MBq)	18 mSv
	Lung ventilation (^{81m}Kr: 6000 MBq)	0.1 mSv
	Cardiac and vascular imaging (^{99m}Tc: 800 MBq)	6 mSv
	Renal imaging (^{123}I: 20 MBq)	0.3 mSv

(see Section 1.8) is invaluable for patient dosimetry during image intensifier screening as the direction of the beam changes during the examination. An ionization chamber can also be used to measure air kerma rate at a given distance from the tube, and an estimate of patient entrance dose can be made from the known exposure factors.

There is a large range in effective dose delivered by different examinations (see Table 6.9). There is also a wide variation in the absorbed dose delivered by a given X-ray examination carried out in different hospitals and sometimes even in the same hospital. Quality assurance has a major role to play in reducing patient dose, as already mentioned.

For nuclear medicine, there is less scope for a wide variation in dose as the maximum activities of radionuclides are determined by the ARSAC. Typical values are given in Section 5.6. Children should be given proportionally less radionuclide, and even so their effective doses may be higher than for adults, and so even greater care needs to be taken.

Entrance surface dose values for a given X-ray examination are up to 100% higher in some hospital departments than in others. The distributions are typical skew (Fig. 6.8), with about 25% of hospitals giving

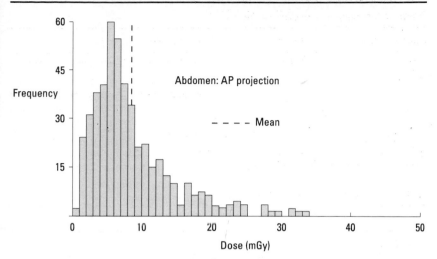

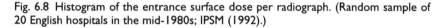

Fig. 6.8 Histogram of the entrance surface dose per radiograph. (Random sample of 20 English hospitals in the mid-1980s; IPSM (1992).)

doses which appear to be unnecessarily high. This 75 percentile value for the dose has been chosen as a reference level in UK diagnostic radiology, both for film radiography (Table 6.10a) and for fluoroscopy. (The data were obtained during the 1980s when the use of rare earth screens was less common. Modern dose reduction techniques should produce a significant decrease in the values of entrance dose and may lead to a downward revision of the reference levels.)

When patient dose measurements (entrance surface dose) are made on a standard-sized (70 kg) patient or using a standard phantom, they should fall below these 75 percentile values for the examination indicated. If this is not the case, the equipment and departmental techniques should be investigated with a view to reducing dose (see Table 6.4) while ensuring good image quality. Similarly, if values below the 10th percentile are measured, the image quality should perhaps be reviewed to ensure it is still of diagnostic value. For details on how to undertake patient dosimetry according to the UK national protocol, see reference IPSM (1992) in the Bibliography. CT dosimetry is discussed in Section 4.3.3.

6.8 PRACTICAL REDUCTION OF DOSE TO STAFF AND VISITORS

Most of the measures which reduce patient dose (Table 6.4) also reduce the dose to staff, and will not be repeated here. X-ray protection to staff has to be provided against the direct beam, leakage radiation, and scatter, particularly from the patient. In nuclear medicine, there are two principal sources – the radionuclide before injection and the patient after injection (see Section 5.7).

Table 6.10a Reference values of entrance surface dose

Site	View	Reference dose (mGy)	
		75 percentile (rounded values)	10 percentile (rounded values)
Lumbar spine	AP	10	4
	Lat	30	10
	LSJ	40	
Abdomen	AP	10	5
Pelvis	AP	10	4
Chest	PA	0.3	0.1
	Lat	1.5	
Skull	AP	5.0	2.0
	PA	5.0	
	Lat	3.0	

AP, anteroposterior; Lat, lateral; LSJ, lumbo-sacral joint; PA, posteroanterior.

Table 6.10b Reference values of the dose–area product

Examination	Reference dose (Gy cm^2) 75 percentile (rounded)
Lumbar spine	15
Barium enema	60
Barium meal	25
Intravenous urography	40
Abdomen	8
Pelvis	5

Sources of X-ray exposure

The direct beam. No-one other than the patient should be exposed to the direct beam. In fluoroscopy the patient should only be palpated on the exit, image intensifier side of the beam. Special care is needed with an overcouch or C-arm tube to avoid putting the hand, head, or forearms into the direct beam. In mobile radiography, special care is needed to avoid exposing anyone, other than the patient, to the direct beam.

Leakage radiation. The tube incorporates lead shielding to attenuate the radiation traveling in any direction other than the useful beam. In whatever way the tube is operated within its rating for an hour, the leakage radiation at a distance of 1 m from the focus must not total more than 1 mSv, and is typically less than 0.1 mSv. The cones, diaphragm, and the housing of the light beam diaphragm afford the same degree of protection. The housing and support plate of the image intensifier have a lead equivalent of typically 2.5 mm.

Scattered radiation. X-rays are scattered in all directions when the X-ray beam strikes any object, including the patient, who is therefore a source of scattered rays whenever the tube is energized. The radiologist and radiographer should be as far away from the patient as practicable for any given procedure. When injecting contrast in CT, it should be remembered that the high kilovoltage used produces a high side scatter. Lead–rubber aprons and curtains, glass screens, etc., should be used to protect staff from scatter. With CT scanners, scatter is high close to the aperture, and this area should be avoided when injecting the patient with contrast medium during exposure.

Reduction of exposure

Distance. The inverse square law affords the cheapest form of protection. Rooms must be adequate in size and no one should stay in the X-ray room (or near the patient in ward radiography) unnecessarily when X-rays are present. There should be no-one in the room during CT warm-up procedures.

In ward radiography, the exposure switch has a cable which allows the operator to stand at least 2 m from the patient. With fixed equipment the switch is normally on the control panel (to prevent the radiographer leaving the protective cubicle during exposure) or at the position of the radiologist.

In interventional procedures, such as catheterization, staff should stand back during exposure unless they have to be near the couch. One large step away usually reduces the dose rate four times. Special care is taken in procedures such as cine angiography which involve several persons, not all of whom are trained radiological staff.

Once nuclear medicine patients have been injected they become sources of exposure to staff. Waiting areas are designed to avoid unnecessary exposure to others. Staff should be able to position and then image the patient with the gamma camera without being unnecessarily exposed.

Speed and time. Reference has already been made to the use of fast recording media and short screening times for patient dose reduction. In fluoroscopy there is a preset timer with a maximum setting of 10 min. (Incidentally, if this were to be reset as many as six times while exposing the same part of the patient, a skin erythema might appear subsequently.) Shorter screening times result in smaller staff doses. Interventional procedures, such as catheterization in which the finger dose may be high, must be carried out expeditiously.

Time spent close to nuclear medicine patients, once injected, should be kept to a reasonable minimum.

Shielding by barriers. Protective barriers should be used when an exposure is made. If this is not practicable, distance and protective clothing should be used. The primary beam must never point toward the protective screen around the control panel as this protects against scatter only. The panel is usually made of plywood incorporating (say) 2.5 mm of lead, which is sufficient to reduce the exposure there, without protective clothing, to the public dose limit. It includes a lead glass window giving a clear view of the patient. See Section 5.7 for the radiopharmacy.

Protective clothing does not protect against the direct beam but only radiation attenuated or scattered by the patient. When palpating, a glove is worn of at least 0.25 mm and preferably 0.35 mm lead equivalent. When injecting, the hands must be outside the direct beam.

Standard body aprons cover some 75% of the red bone marrow and are not less than 0.25 mm lead equivalent (which typically transmits only 10% of 90° scatter). In interventional radiology, aprons should cover as large an area as possible and have a front of 0.35 or 0.5 mm lead equivalent. Aprons are provided in all X-ray rooms and with each mobile set. They must be stored carefully without folding, e.g. draped over a thick rail, to avoid cracking. They are examined periodically using X-rays to check for cracks.

Thyroid protection shields are also recommended to be worn during fluoroscopic procedures. Lead glass spectacles may be worn during some interventional procedures, or a pull-down lead glass window may be used.

In fluoroscopy with an undercouch tube, sufficiently large drapes of 0.5 mm lead equivalent are attached to the lower edge of the image intensifier when the table or stand is vertical, and to the operator's side when it is horizontal.

Special care must be taken in fluoroscopy and interventional procedures, particularly cine angiography, all of which are liable to expose staff to high doses. Thin lead protection, adequate for X-rays, is insufficient for the higher energies in *gamma imaging*. In this case, distance and time are important factors for staff dose reduction when the patient is the source.

Warning lights and signs

On the X-ray control panel a light comes on when the set is switched on. Another light comes on when the tube is energized, and stays on long enough to be noticed, even if the exposure is brief.

On or close to each tube housing, when more than one tube can be energized from a single control position, yellow or amber lights come on when the tube is selected.

At the entrance to the X-ray room there is a warning sign to indicate a 'controlled area' due to X-rays and a warning light which comes on during fluoroscopy and when the tube is 'prepared' for radiography.

In nuclear medicine, warning signs alone are adequate. Warning lights are not deemed helpful as the hazard is effectively present all the time.

Protection of the public

X-ray rooms are shielded through their walls, windows, and doors to reduce the dose in surrounding areas below the levels for 'other persons', i.e. 0.1 mSv per week^{-1} under normal workloads. The doors, windows, and the greater part of the walls only receive scattered rays, and some 2.5 mm lead equivalent is often satisfactory. The protection is greater in areas of the walls and floors where the direct beam may fall. The protection needed is first calculated in terms of lead and then realized as an equivalent combination of other materials. By way of illustration, the following are approximately equal in their protective power for diagnostic X-rays:

120 mm of concrete

12 mm of barium plaster

1 mm of lead

Radiopharmacies are similarly protected, and consideration has to be given to visitors in nuclear medicine waiting areas.

Supporting children during radiography

If possible, restraining and supporting devices are used to hold children or infirm patients during radiography. If this is not practicable, children may be supported by an accompanying adult, although preferably not by a woman known to be pregnant. He or she is instructed how to do so, is positioned outside the beam, and wears a protective apron or is otherwise shielded by a barrier. A direct-reading radiation monitor may provide reassurance.

6.9 PERSONAL DOSIMETRY SYSTEMS

Three different personal dosimetry systems will be described. Their relative advantages or disadvantages are summarized in Table 6.11.

6.9.1 Film badges

Personal monitoring film is exposed without screens, inside an appropriate holder. It is usually the same size as a dental film, sometimes smaller.

It is double coated: one emulsion is slow, and is relatively unaffected by normal occupational doses; the other emulsion is fast, and its blackening is used to assess normal occupational doses. High (accidental and emergency) doses will completely blacken the fast emulsion so that they cannot be assessed with accuracy. Removing an area of this emulsion (with a damp swab) reveals the lesser blackening of the slow emulsion, which allows the high dose to be assessed.

Monitoring films are placed in a plastic cassette or 'badge' which may be pinned to the clothing, can carry an identification of the wearer, and, most importantly, incorporates plastic and metal filters, to differentiate the radiations received (Fig. 6.9a).

Each month the requisite number of films from a single manufacturing batch (and therefore of closely similar sensitivities) are stamped with identifying serial numbers (which can been seen through the open window in the badge). A proportion of these are retained in the laboratory as calibration films (or 'standards').

Personal dosemeters are usually calibrated by exposure to a series of known doses of gamma rays from a radioactive source with a long half-life, such as the 662 keV gamma rays from ^{137}Cs.

After they have been worn for a month, the dosemeters are returned to the approved dosimetry laboratory, where the films are all processed under carefully controlled conditions.

The densities of the calibration films are measured, and a graph is plotted of density of blackening under a lead filter versus dose. The densities of the films worn by personnel are then measured, and the doses apparently received are read from the appropriate calibration curve.

The film dosemeter is *energy-dependent* because silver and bromine have much higher atomic numbers than tissue or air. To produce the same

Table 6.11 Personal dosimetry systems: advantages and disadvantages

Advantages	Disadvantages
Film badges	
Relatively cheap	Requires dark room and wet
Permanent record of the exposure	processing
Wide range of dose (0.2–1000 mSv)	Lower threshold for hard gamma
Identifies type and energy of exposure	radiation is 0.15 mSv
Easy to identify individual dosemeters	Is affected by heat, humidity, and
	chemicals
Thermoluminescent (TL) personal dosemeters	
Chips can be reused	Requires a high capital outlay
Wide range of dose (0.1–2000 mSv)	No permanent record (other than
Direct reading of personal dose	glow curves)
Energy independent within ±10%	Cannot distinguish radioactive
Compact: suitable for finger dosimetry	contamination
	Requires a filtered badge to provide
	energy discrimination
Siemens electronic personal dosemeter (EPD)	
Direct reading and cumulative	Initial cost
record storage (up to 16 Sv)	Linear response to dose
Flat response: 20 keV to 10 MeV	Is quite heavy, but weighs less than a
Can be 'zeroed' by user without	hospital 'bleep'
deleting cumulative record	Battery should be renewed each year
Measures personal dose at depth	
and at the skin directly, to 1 μSv	
Audible warning of high dose rates	

blackening requires exposure to increasing amounts of the following radiations:

◆ low-energy scattered rays;
◆ direct rays from a diagnostic X-ray tube;
◆ gamma rays from ^{99m}Tc; and the
◆ gamma rays from ^{137}Cs used for calibration.

For example, diagnostic X-rays produce about 10 times the blackening as the same absorbed dose of gamma rays from diagnostic radionuclides.

Particularly when a film is worn by someone exposed to *mixed* radiations – direct diagnostic X-rays, scattered X-rays, and energetic gamma rays from radionuclides, for example – an analysis has to be made of the various energy components.

To identify the various components, the film badge sandwiches the film

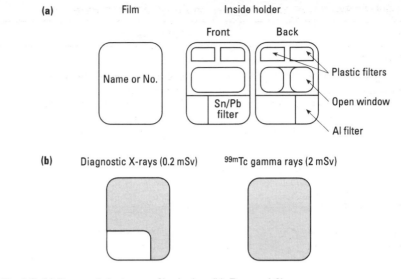

Fig. 6.9 (a) Personal dosimetry film badge. (b) Exposed films.

between at least three pairs of *filters*: (a) 'thick plastic', (b) aluminum, and (c) tin with a thin lead foil (Fig. 6.9a).

Roughly speaking, high-energy photons are somewhat attenuated by the tin–lead filter but not by the other two. Medium-energy scatter from a diagnostic X-ray tube is heavily attenuated by the tin–lead filter, is somewhat attenuated by the aluminum, but not by the plastic. Low-energy scattered radiation does not penetrate either of the metal filters.

As a result, the appearance of the film shows a pattern of the shadows of the three filters and gives an indication of the type(s) of radiation to which it has been exposed (Fig. 6.9b). The dose of mixed radiations can be evaluated from the film densities measured under each of the filters using the relative speed of the film to radiations of different energies, and the calibration curve.

In addition, a sharp edge to the shadows of the filters suggests a single exposure to direct rays from one direction; a blurred edge that exposure has been to scattered rays or many small exposures from different directions. Spots of intense blackening suggest a radioactive spill.

The film badge can also measure *other kinds of ionizing radiations*. There are one or more thin plastic filters as well as the thick one. These together with the open window (no filter) allow the dose of beta rays of various ranges or energies to be assessed. In some types of badge there is an additional filter of cadmium, which allows the dose from slow neutrons to be assessed separately.

6.9.2 Thermoluminescent dosemeters

These are available in many different forms and materials. In one simple form a small chip of lithium fluoride is mounted in a plastic holder which carries identifying details and is pinned to the wearer. As with any phosphor, when X- or gamma rays fall on lithium fluoride and are absorbed, atomic electrons are raised to higher energy levels. In the case of a thermoluminescent (TL) material such as lithium fluoride the electrons stay indefinitely in their excited state (in 'electron traps'), and the material retains a 'memory' of the radiation exposure. The greater the dose absorbed, the more electrons are 'trapped'. After the badge has been worn for the prescribed period it is returned to the approved dosimetry laboratory where it is processed.

The chip of TL material is inserted in a light-tight chamber, and its temperature is raised to 300–400°C at a carefully controlled rate. This causes the trapped electrons to leave the traps and fall to their ground state. In doing so they emit photons of light which are collected and measured by a photoelectric device as the temperature is raised ('glow curve'). The total light energy emitted under the curve is proportional to the dose of X- or gamma rays originally absorbed. Calibration is performed as with film dosemeters. The dose is indicated on a digital read-out, and may be digitized and stored in a computer, together with the glow curve of the TL material characterized by the dose received.

The chip is then annealed using another controlled heating program to remove any residual stored energy and any 'memory' of the previous exposure. Having been returned to its original condition, it can then be reissued for reuse.

In other forms, TL dosemeters are also used to measure patient dose in radiological procedures; mounted in rings to measure staff finger doses; or, in sachets, placed on the forehead to estimate eye doses.

6.9.3 Electronic dosemeters

Direct-reading electronic dosemeters based on Geiger-Müller tubes or single silicon diodes can provide effective alarms and immediate dose readings in areas where there are real risks of high exposures. However, these devices have a very poor response to photon energies below around 80 keV. This makes them unable to detect low-energy gamma radiation and diagnostic X-rays. The Siemens electronic personal dosemeter (EPD) overcomes that problem with a linear response to below 20 keV, which makes it suitable for radiodiagnostic staff. To date, the EPD has achieved approval as a legal personal dosemeter in the UK, Norway, Italy and Germany.

The EPD was developed by Siemens in conjunction with the UK National Radiological Protection Board (NRPB) using two silicon photodiodes to overcome the energy response limitations of a single detector. The read-out display gives the personal equivalent dose to the body and also to the skin. It can also indicate dose rates with or without an alarm feature. The stored doses can be read out using a special reader coupled to a computer to record the values in an individual dose record. The information includes the time when significant dose rates were recorded, which can help in tracing potential incidents. The sensitivity is 50–200 times greater than that of a TLD. This makes it highly appropriate for measuring doses in diagnostic imaging where individual doses are low and where the proposed limits on a *pro rata* monthly basis (0.15 mSv) for pregnant workers would be difficult to assure with either films or a TLD.

A major advantage of such a direct reading dosemeter is that each wearer can see when and where doses are being accrued and can take appropriate steps to reduce exposure. A disadvantage is its initial cost (about £300) but as its life is expected to be 10 years, the effective monthly cost is on a par with most TLD or commercial film systems. The battery only needs to be replaced every 12 months, at which time a calibration check is recommended. The EPD is calibrated for 'life' when manufactured, but an annual check may be needed to comply with legal approval.

6.10 BIBLIOGRAPHY OF OFFICIAL DOCUMENTS

1 ICRP 60 (1991) 1991 Recommendations of the International Commission on Radiological Protection. *Annals of the ICRP*, **21**, Nos. 1–3. Pergamon Press, Oxford.
2 RCR (1995) *Making the Best Use of the Radiology Department*, 3rd edn. Royal College of Radiologists, London.
3 IRR (1985) *Ionising Radiations Regulations (1985)*, No. 1333. HMSO, London.
4 IRR (1988) *Ionising Radiation (Protection of Persons Undergoing Medical Examination or Treatment) Regulations (1988)*. HMSO, London.
5 IRR (1988) *Ionising Radiation (Protection of Patients) Regulations 1988 (Northern Ireland)*. HMSO, Northern Ireland.
6 RSA (1993) *Radioactive Substances Act (1993)*, HMSO, London.
7 ACOP (1985) The protection of persons against ionising radiation arising from any work activity. *Ionising Radiations Regulations, Approved Code of Practice*. HMSO, London.
8 ACOP Part 4 (1991) *Ionising Radiations Regulations, Approved Code of Practice Part 4*. HMSO, London.
9 Guidance Note (1988) *Guidance Notes for the Protection of Persons Against Ionising Radiations Arising from Medical and Dental Use*. NRPB, Oxon.
10 ARSAC (1993) *Notes for Guidance on the Administration of Radioactive Substances to Persons for Purposes of Diagnosis, Treatment or Research*. Administration of Radioactive Substances Advisory Committee, Department of Health, London.
11 Guidance Note PM77 (1992) *Fitness of Equipment used for Medical Exposure to Ionising Radiation*. HSE, London.
12 HSG (91) 11 (1991) *Patient Dose-Reduction: Purchasing Radiology Equipment*. NHS Medical Devices Directorate, London.
13 IPSM (1992) *National Protocol for Patient Dose Measurements in Diagnostic Radiology*. NRPB, Oxon.

VIVA QUESTIONS

1. How do X- and gamma radiations damage cells?

2. What methods of personal dosimetry are there?

3. Compare and contrast the film badge with a thermoluminescent dosemeter (TLD) or an electronic dosemeter (EPD).

4. What is a classified person and what are the legal requirements?

5. What are the dose limits for (a) classified workers, (b) other workers, and (c) members of the public?

6. What steps would you take to minimize patient dosage from (a) a barium meal, (b) a CT abdominal scan, and (c) a pelvic radiograph?

7. What methods of radiation protection are available for members of staff within a radiology department?

8. What is a controlled area and what are the legal requirements?

9. Explain the need for the '28-day rule'.

10. Explain the terms (a) effective dose and (b) tissue weighting factor.

11. What are the differences between stochastic and deterministic effects of radiation?

12. What are 'local' rules?

13. What is meant by the 'core of knowledge' as detailed in the 1988 POPUMET regulations?

14. What are the dangers to the fetus of X-radiation and how do they differ during development?

15. What are the reference doses for (a) a chest X-ray, (b) an intravenous urogram, (c) a barium enema, (d) a CT head scan, and (e) a ^{99m}Tc bone image? How do these relate to effective doses received by a patient?

7

IMAGING WITH ULTRASOUND

Ultrasound refers to sound waves of such a high frequency (above 20 kHz) as to be inaudible to humans. Whereas audible sound spreads through a room, ultrasound with its shorter wavelength can be formed into a narrow beam, though not as well as light with its even shorter wavelength.

Ultrasound, although not electromagnetic radiation, undergoes reflection and refraction at the interface between two different media. It is such reflections or echoes from different tissues that produce the ultrasound images. Diagnostic ultrasound has a special place in imaging soft tissues that are too similar to produce enough X-ray contrast; and also in obstetric imaging, as the hazards are perceived to be insignificant compared with X-rays.

Ultrasound waves are produced by a transducer which consists primarily of a piezoceramic disk or rectangular plate. This is made of compressed microcrystalline lead zirconate titanate (PZT) or of the plastic polyvinylidine difluoride (PVDF). The two flat faces are made electrically conducting with a very thin coating of silver.

7.1 PIEZOELECTRIC EFFECT

When a direct (DC) voltage is applied to the flat faces of the disk it expands (or contracts), and if the voltage is reversed it contracts (or expands). The movement of the faces is proportional to the voltage.

183

When the disk is compressed, equal and opposite charges and a corresponding voltage appear on the two flat faces; if the pressure is reversed, so is the voltage. The voltage produced is proportional to the pressure.

When an alternating voltage is applied, the disk alternately expands and contracts with the same frequency.

When the disk is subjected to an alternating pressure, an alternating voltage is produced of the same frequency.

The same transducer will convert electrical into sound energy and vice versa, and can act as both a transmitter and a receiver.

When heated above a certain temperature (about 350°C for PZT), called its *Curie temperature*, transducers lose their piezoelectric properties. Transducer probes should obviously not be autoclaved (nor should they be immersed in water unless waterproofed). Thin slices of naturally occurring quartz crystals also show the piezoelectric effect, and are used in digital timers and computers.

Transducers are used in both pulsed and continuous-wave modes.

Pulsed mode

When the transducer is in contact with a patient (or some other medium) and a few hundred volts DC are suddenly applied to the disk, it instantly expands, thereby compressing a layer of the material in contact with it (Fig. 7.1a). Due to the elasticity of the material the compressed layer expands and compresses an adjacent layer of material (Fig. 7.1b). In this way a layer or wave of compression travels with a velocity v through the material, followed by a corresponding wave of decompression or rarefaction. In imaging, such short regular pulses of ultrasound are used.

Continuous-wave mode

If instead an alternating (AC) voltage is applied, the crystal face pulses forward and backward like a piston, producing successive compressions

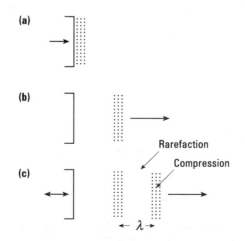

Fig. 7.1 Production of sound waves by a transducer.

and rarefactions (Fig. 7.1c). Each compression wave has moved forward a distance called the *wavelength* (λ) by the time the next one is produced.

The *frequency* (f) with which compressions pass any given point is the same as the frequency at which the transducer vibrates and the frequency of the AC voltage applied to it. It is measured in megahertz (MHz).

The density and therefore the pressure of the material rises and falls above its normal value (of 1 atm, 101 kPa). In a typical diagnostic application the particles travel to and fro through distances less than 1 μm, with velocities up to 500 mm s^{-1} and accelerations up to 300 000g. The peak of the pressure wave can reach several atmospheres.

The graph of pressure excess p at any point against time t is a sine wave (Fig. 7.2a), the interval between successive crests being the period $T = 1/f$. A graph of pressure excess at any instant t_1 against distance d through the material is also sinusoidal (solid curve in Fig. 7.2b), the distance between successive crests being the wavelength λ. The dashed curve refers to a later

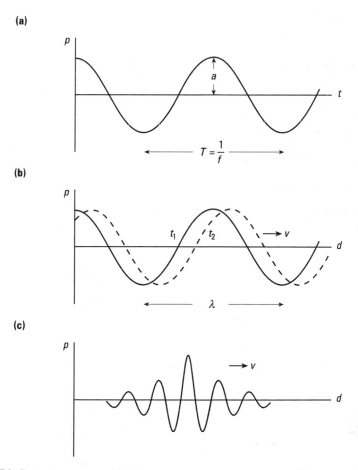

Fig. 7.2 Excess pressure: (a) versus time: continuous wave; (b) versus distance: continuous wave; (c) versus distance: pulsed wave.

instant t_2. The wave travels forward with a velocity v. As with any sine wave,

$$\text{wavelength} \times \text{frequency} = \text{velocity}$$

or

$$\lambda f = v$$

For comparison, Fig. 7.2c shows the pressure waveform of a pulsed wave, a few periods in duration.

Properties of ultrasound

Unlike light and X-rays, sound requires a material medium in which to travel, and is a longitudinal, not a transverse, wave. Unlike X- and gamma rays, it can be reflected, refracted, and focused, and its wavelength is sufficiently long for its wave properties (interference and diffraction) to predominate. Unlike light, its velocity in matter is, for practical purposes, independent of frequency.

The *velocity* of ultrasound depends on the material through which it travels. The greater the density, the lower the velocity. The greater the compressibility (or the smaller the elastic modulus), the lower the velocity. Accordingly, velocity depends on temperature.

Some typical figures are given in the first two columns of Table 7.1. Note that sound takes nearly 7 μs to travel each centimeter in average soft tissue. The table also lists the product of velocity and density, called the acoustic impedance, as explained in Section 7.4.

Air has a much lower density but it is much more compressible than water or tissue; hence the low velocity.

Since the frequency of a given transducer is fixed, wavelength is proportional to velocity. If a transducer is energized at a frequency of 3.5 MHz, the wavelength of the ultrasound changes as it travels from the transducer (1 mm) through soft tissue (0.4 mm) to bone (0.9 mm).

The intensity of ultrasound, measured in watts per square millimeter (W mm^{-2}), is proportional to the square of the wave amplitude (a in Fig. 7.2a), and is under the operator's control.

7.2 INTERFERENCE

If two sound waves of the same wavelength cross each other the pressure waves combine. If, as in Fig. 7.3a, the two waves, A and B, are exactly in step (in phase) their amplitudes add up; this is called constructive

Table 7.1 Velocity of ultrasound in various materials

	Velocity (m s^{-1})	Density (kg m^{-3})	Acoustic impedance Z (kg m^{-2} s^{-1})
Air	330	1.29	430
Average soft tissue[1]	1540	1000	1.5 million
Typical bone	3200	1650	5.3 million
PZT	4000	7500	30 million

[1]Range of velocity: 1300 to 1800 m s^{-1}

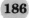
186

(a)

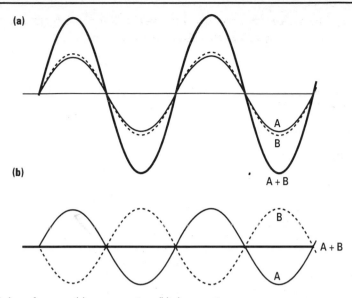

(b)

Fig. 7.3 Interference: (a) constructive; (b) destructive.

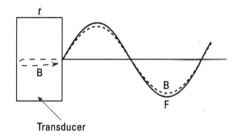

Fig. 7.4 Resonance.

interference. If, as in Fig. 7.3b, they are exactly out of step (180° out of phase) they tend to cancel each other out; this is called destructive interference. If they are only partially out of step, they result in a wave of reduced intensity.

Natural or resonant frequency

A transducer can be made to emit sound of any frequency by driving it (in continuous mode) with AC of that frequency. However, a transducer vibrates most violently and produces the largest output of sound when the frequency at which it is made to vibrate produces a wavelength in the transducer equal to twice the thickness (t) of the piezoelectric disk, for the following reason.

In Fig. 7.4 the front face of the transducer emits sound both in the forward and backward directions. The back wave B is reflected at the back face of the disk. By the time it joins the front wave F, it has travelled an

187

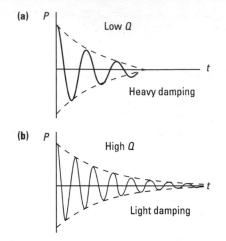

Fig. 7.5 Damping: (a) heavy; (b) light.

extra distance $2t$. If, as in the diagram, this equals a wavelength (or any exact number of wavelengths) the F and B waves reinforce, for they are exactly in phase. Constructive interference or resonance occurs. Otherwise there will be some destructive interference.

The frequency at which the transducer is the most efficient as a transmitter of sound is also the frequency at which it is most sensitive as a receiver of sound. It is called its natural or resonant frequency.

However, if the same transducer disk is made to vibrate by striking it, or by suddenly and briefly applying a large DC voltage (in pulse mode), it vibrates at its natural frequency. It will emit sound of a frequency which has a wavelength of $2t$. Sound of any other frequency would very quickly die away due to destructive interference, in the manner described above. The thicker the crystal the lower the natural frequency and the longer the wavelength. The transducer has a natural period $T = 1/f$.

The *natural or resonant frequency* of a transducer disk depends on (a) its dimensions, particularly its thickness, and (b) its material, which affects the velocity of sound in it. To change the frequency one has to change the transducer. A 3.5 MHz transducer has a crystal some 0.5 mm thick.

Pulse duration or length

Once the transducer has been pulsed, it continues to vibrate for a short while with diminishing amplitude as it loses energy in the form of sound. As shown in Fig. 7.5, the amplitude of the pressure wave decays exponentially with time. This is called *damping*. If the vibrations continue for an appreciable period it is called 'ringing'. If the damping is heavy (Fig. 7.5a), it has a short time constant or 'ring-down time'. It is said to have a low 'quality factor' (Q), defined below. A transducer which is more lightly damped has a higher Q and, as in Fig. 7.5b, produces a longer pulse and a higher output of sound.

Typically, the duration of the ultrasound pulse may be three periods or less (about 1 μs with a 3.5 MHz transducer). The pulse length can equally well be stated as three wavelengths or less (about 1.5 mm in tissue).

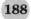

Ultrasound travels at a nominally constant speed in tissue, so time and distance can often be used interchangeably.

7.3 SINGLE TRANSDUCER PROBE

Figure 7.6 illustrates the essential features of a single transducer, as used in a mechanical sector scanner (see Section 7.8). In the transmitting mode, the energizing voltage is applied between the back face of the piezoelectric disk (3) via an insulated wire (1), and the front face via an earthed metal case (2).

The back face is cemented to a 'backing block' (4) of epoxy resin in which are suspended fine particles of tungsten. The backing block and transducer are 'matched', as described in Section 7.4, so as to admit the backward-traveling waves produced by the back face of the vibrating disk. These waves are scattered and absorbed within the block. Like a tympanist placing a hand on a drum face, this damps the vibration. It results in a short pulse and a low Q. Additional damping and further shortening of the pulse is performed electronically by applying a second reverse, voltage pulse very shortly after the first. If the block is omitted, so that the disk is backed with air, total reflection takes place, the pulse lasts for 20 or more periods, and the Q and the sound output are increased.

The front face of the disk is fixed to a thin plastic slip (5), which, as well as protecting the surface of the disk, has other important properties (see Section 7.4). In the receiving mode, the signal voltage produced by the returning echo is led away along a wire (1).

Bandwidth

In continuous mode the transducer emits sound of a single frequency. The frequency spectrum, which plots relative intensity against frequency of sound, is a single line (a in Fig. 7.7). In pulsed mode it emits a continuous spectrum (b and c in Fig. 7.7) of sine waves having a limited range of frequencies, which combine to form the pulse. The bandwidth is the full width at half maximum intensity (FWHM) of the frequency spectrum. A short pulse (c) has a wider bandwidth of frequencies than a longer pulse (b).

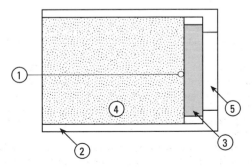

Fig. 7.6 Section through a single transducer probe.

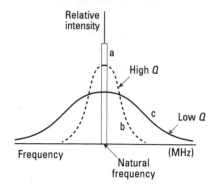

Fig. 7.7 Frequency spectrum in (a) continuous and (b,c) pulsed modes.

The same graphs (b and c) represent the 'resonance curve', the response of the transducer as a receiver to waves of different frequencies. The *quality factor (Q)*, referred to above, is the ratio of mean frequency to bandwidth. The greater Q, the narrower the bandwidth both as transmitter and receiver. A transducer with a high Q produces a pure note and responds only to that note. One with a low Q has a short ring-down time, produces short pulses and responds to a band of frequencies.

Diameter of the transducer

If the transducer had a diameter equal to one wavelength or less (say 0.5 mm), sound would spread out equally in all directions, as spherical waves, and would have no directional properties. This is shown in Fig. 7.8a, in which dashed lines represent wavefronts and the solid lines, rays showing the direction of propagation of the waves.

If, as in Fig. 7.8b, its diameter D is, for example, 10 times the wavelength, sound is projected forward effectively as a plane wave, in a beam of approximately the same diameter as the transducer, for the following reason.

Imagine that the face of the disk is subdivided into 80 small transducers, each 0.5 mm in size, all emitting waves at the same time. For every crest that reaches any point B outside the beam from one minitransducer, a trough arrives simultaneously from another minitransducer, and there is (more or less) total destructive interference of the sound. The separate sound waves that similarly reach any point A inside the beam are, in the main, roughly in phase, and they reinforce each other by constructive interference.

Near and far fields

As a result of the interference described above, the sound energy is largely confined to the beam of diameter D. The nearly parallel part of the beam N is called the near field or the Fresnel region, and extends a distance $D^2/4\lambda$ from the transducer face. In other words, the length of the near zone is proportional to fD^2.

At greater depths in F, the far field or the Fraunhofer region, the interference effect is lost and the beam diverges. The angle of divergence θ increases as λ/D increases. In other words, the far zone divergence

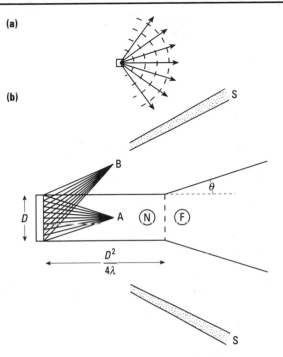

(a)

(b)

Fig. 7.8 Pattern of sound emitted by (a) a very small transducer element and (b) a larger diameter transducer (near and far fields).

increases as fD decreases. Due to vibration of the edges of the transducer disk, there are small beams of low intensity outside the beam in what are called 'side lobes' (S in Fig. 7.8). They may cause image artefacts.

For example, at a frequency of 3.5 MHz, a 12 mm diameter transducer has a near field 80 mm in depth and a divergence angle of between 1 and 2°.

Using a transducer of higher frequency increases the length of the near zone and decreases the divergence of the far zone (for the same diameter of disk). The beam becomes more directional – just, as in stereo equipment, the tweeter is more directional than the woofer.

Using a transducer of larger diameter increases the length of the near zone and decreases the divergence of the far zone (for the same frequency).

Focusing

Transducers may be designed to focus at a particular depth (or, rather, range of depths) corresponding to the region of diagnostic interest. This concentrates its intensity so that it will produce stronger echoes and improves its lateral resolution. There are several ways to focus the beam:

◆ Using a *curved* (concave, spherical) piezoelectric element. The shape of the beam is sketched in Fig. 7.9. Being a ceramic it can be molded into any shape. The greater the curvature, the shorter the focal length.

◆ Using a plastic *acoustic lens* cemented to the transducer face in Fig. 7.6). (This converging lens will be concave or convex according to its material.) Sometimes a curved mirror is used instead.

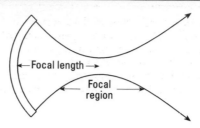

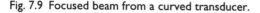

Fig. 7.9 Focused beam from a curved transducer.

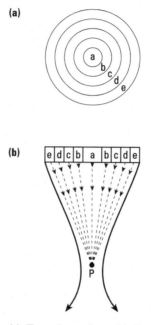

Fig. 7.10 Annular array. (a) Transducer face. (b) Cross section through the transducer and the ultrasound beam.

Transducers can be made with strong, intermediate or weak focusing. The price of a short focal length is increased divergence of the far field. The shorter the focal length, the narrower and shorter the focal region or 'depth of focus', over which the beam is reasonably narrow, as depicted in Fig. 7.9.

◆ *Electronic focusing: annular array*, used in mechanical sector scanners.

Figure 7.10a shows the face of a circular piezoelectric disk subdivided into five concentric rings a, b, c, d and e. If they were all energized simultaneously, they would act as a single transducer, and the resulting beam would have the shape depicted in Fig. 7.8b.

If however the outermost ring (e) is energized first, the next ring (d) a very little later, then subsequent rings (c and b), and finally the central element (a), there will be a point P at which the pulses, traveling along paths of different lengths, all arrive together and so reinforce. The resulting beam shape is shown in Fig. 7.10b, the energy being concentrated or focused in the region of P. In compensation, the beam diverges more at greater depths.

The focal length can be altered without changing the transducer: the greater the time delays between energizing successive annular rings, the shorter the focal length. Electronic focusing is considered further in Section 7.8.

7.4 BEHAVIOR OF A BEAM AT AN INTERFACE BETWEEN DIFFERENT MATERIALS

If a beam strikes the boundary between two materials (transducer–skin, tissue–bone, tissue–air, etc.) at right angles, some of the energy is reflected as an 'echo' and some is transmitted.

Acoustic impedance

The proportions of energy reflected and transmitted depend on the acoustic impedances of the two materials. The acoustic impedance (Z) of a material is defined as the product of the density (ρ) of the material and the velocity (v) of sound in it. It is for practical purposes independent of frequency. Some values are given in SI units in the third column of Table 7.1.

$Z = v\rho$, and therefore depends on the density and elasticity of the material.

The fraction of sound energy that is reflected at the interface between two materials depends on the angle of incidence. When the beam strikes the surface at or nearly at right angles, the fraction of sound energy that is reflected at the interface between two materials of acoustic impedances Z_1 and Z_2 is

$$\text{reflected fraction } R = \frac{(Z_1 - Z_2)^2}{(Z_1 + Z_2)^2}$$

It is the same whether the sound is traveling from material 1 to material 2 or vice versa. The greater the difference in acoustic impedance the greater the fraction R reflected. The less the difference in acoustic impedance, the greater $(1 - R)$, the fraction transmitted. In consequence:

◈ When $Z_1 = Z_2$ there is 100% transmission and no reflection. The two materials are said to be acoustically 'matched' as, for example, the transducer and the backing block (see Section 7.3).

◈ At an interface between bone ($Z = 5$ million) and tissue ($Z = 1.5$ million) the fraction reflected is

$$(5.0 - 1.5)^2/(5.0 + 1.5)^2$$

or about 30%. About 70% of the sound energy is therefore transmitted. Generally speaking, it is not possible to image through bone.

◈ At any interface with air or gas (Z negligible) total reflection occurs, with the following results:

(a) Gas-filled organs cast a shadow, and structures underneath cannot be imagined. Normal lung cannot be penetrated. The bowel wall can be visualized but not the lumen itself. Ultrasound is sometimes used to check for air in vessels, e.g. within the liver.

Table 7.2. Acoustic impedances of different tissues

Tissue	Acoustic impedance $(kg\ m^{-2}\ s^{-1})$
Fat	1.38×10^6
Kidney	1.62×10^6
Liver	1.64×10^6
Muscle	1.70×10^6
Spleen	1.63×10^6

Table 7.3. Typical reflection factors

Interface	Percentage
Gas–tissue	99.9
Bone–muscle	30
Fat–muscle	1
Blood–muscle	0.1
Liver–muscle	0.01
Soft tissue–PZT	80
Plastic–soft tissue	10

(b) It is impossible to get sound from the transducer to the patient and vice versa if there is air trapped between the transducer and the skin; it is all reflected back. For this reason the transducer is pressed against the patient and a coupling oil or gel is used. Bubbles of air must be avoided.

◆ Because of the 'mismatch' of acoustic impedance between transducer and tissue, only some 20% of the sound energy would be transmitted in either direction between the transducer and the patient. This is overcome by attaching to the front face of the transducer a *matching plate* (5 in Fig. 7.6) a quarter of a wavelength thick and made of a plastic compound having an acoustic impedance intermediate between that of the transducer and the skin – as close as possible to the geometric mean.

◆ The figures given so far for 'tissue' refer to average soft tissue. There are subtle differences of density, elasticity, and, therefore, acoustic impedance between different soft tissues (Table 7.2).

Small fractions of ultrasound are therefore reflected at interfaces between different soft tissues, e.g. nearly 1% at a fat–kidney interface. Approximate values are given in Table 7.3. Reflections less than 0.01% are unlikely to be detected.

Specular (mirror) reflection

If a beam strikes a large smooth interface at an angle, the same laws of reflection and refraction apply as with light (Fig. 7.11a):

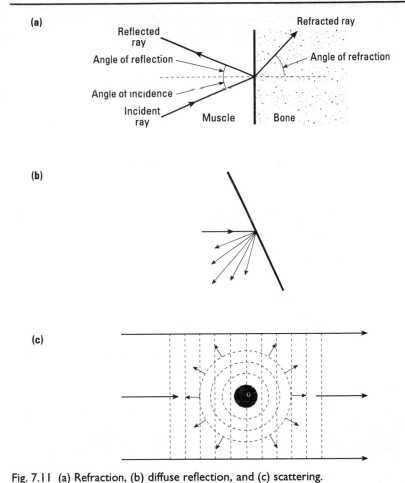

Fig. 7.11 (a) Refraction, (b) diffuse reflection, and (c) scattering.

- the angle of reflection = the angle of incidence;
- the ratio

$$\frac{\text{sine of the angle of incidence}}{\text{sine of the angle of refraction}}$$

is equal to the ratio

$$\frac{\text{velocity of sound in the first material}}{\text{velocity of sound in the second material}}$$

This is Snell's law.

Diffuse reflection

If, as is usually the case, the tissue interface is 'rough' and has undulations equal to a wavelength or so, the reflected beam spread out over an angle

(Fig. 7.11b). The same effect is seen with light and frosted glass. The shorter the wavelength and also the rougher the surface, the wider the spread. On account of this, in imaging, the transducer will receive some reflections even if the beam does not strike an interface exactly at right angles.

Scatter

When sound encounters a structure that is much smaller than a wavelength (such as a red blood corpuscle, diameter 10 μm, or tissue parenchyma) it is reradiated more or less equally in all directions. This is shown in Fig. 7.11c, in which dashed lines represent wavefronts, and solid lines, rays. This effect allows even small structures to be visualized, as some scatter will reach the transducer. The echo signals so produced from the interior of the placenta, liver, pancreas, spleen, and kidney are about 1/10 or 1/100 as strong as those produced by the organ boundaries. Scattering by red blood cells, on which blood flow imaging depends, produces even smaller signals, and so necessitates a high frequency (see Section 7.13).

7.5 ATTENUATION OF ULTRASOUND

When traveling through a material, sound is attenuated exponentially with the depth of travel for the following reasons:

◈ Energy is absorbed (and converted into heat) by frictional and viscous forces in the material.
◈ Energy leaves the forward-traveling beam due to scattering, and to partial reflection by the multitude of interfaces that the beam encounters *en route*. The higher the frequency, the greater the attenuation.

Attenuation is measured in decibels (dB) (see Section 7.16). In average tissue, sound of frequency 1 MHz loses about 1 dB cm^{-1}, corresponding to a half value layer (HVL) of about 3 cm. The decibel loss per centimeter is proportional to the frequency. Thus, at 3.5 MHz the loss is about 3.5 dB cm^{-1}. In a journey to and fro through 15 cm depth of tissue the total loss would then be 100 dB. In water and blood there is little absorption or scatter. In certain circumstances a full bladder can aid penetration. In bone the attenuation is greater: 35 dB cm^{-1} at 2.5 MHz. Air attenuates heavily: in lung, attenuation is 40 dB cm^{-1} MHz^{-1}.

Penetration

At a certain depth the intensity of the beam has fallen too low to be useful. The higher the frequency produced by the transducer, the less the effective penetration of the beam. Roughly, *penetration (cm) = 40/frequency (MHz)*.

7.6 A-MODE (AMPLITUDE MODE–ECHORANGING)

A-mode imaging is sometimes used for examining the eye or for showing mid-line displacement in the brain. It is the simplest form of ultrasound imaging which shows only the position of tissue interfaces. As an imaging technique it has been largely superseded by B-mode imaging or other

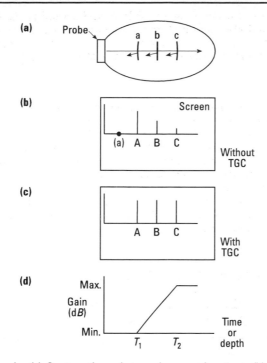

Fig. 7.12 A-mode. (a) Section through transducer and patient. (b) Trace on screen without time gain control. (c) Trace on screen using time gain control. (d) Variation of swept gain with depth.

imaging techniques, such as computed tomography (CT). However, A-mode illustrates the basic principles of ultrasound imaging.

The probe is held stationary against the patient (Fig. 7.12a). It is pulsed (with a voltage of a few hundred volts lasting for a few nanoseconds) and simultaneously the light spot starts to move from the left hand edge of the monitor screen (Fig. 7.12b). While the pulse of ultrasound travels with a velocity averaging 1.5 mm μs^{-1} through the patient, the light spot moves at a constant speed, tracing out a horizontal line across the screen.

It takes the ultrasound pulse a time t to reach interface a, by which time the light spot has reached point a on the screen. Some of the energy is reflected back along the path as an 'echo' pulse, which takes a further time t to return to the probe, by which time the light spot has reached 'A'.

The probe now acts as a receiver and, in response to the echo received, generates a small signal voltage which, after amplification, produces, at A, a short vertical trace ('blip') of height proportional to the echo strength. The other interfaces b and c each produce blips at B and C, respectively. The locations of the blips along the trace indicate the depths of the corresponding interfaces along the beam. A 'clock' can be used to superimpose on the horizontal trace a ruler or caliper – a sequence of marker pulses spaced to correspond to 1 cm intervals in the body.

To provide a sustained image the pulse is repeated, typically 1000 times a second (*the pulse repetition frequency* (PRF) is 1 kHz). After the transducer has been pulsed for about 1 μs (transmit mode) it is then available to receive echoes (receive or listening mode) for about 999 μs before it is pulsed again.

Time gain compensation

Due to attenuation in the tissue, the amplitude of the sound pulse diminishes as it travels into the body, and the echo pulse is similarly attenuated as it travels back toward the transducer. A particular interface, or 'reflector', deep in the body therefore produces a much weaker echo than an identical interface near the surface, as seen in Fig. 7.12b.

Attenuation is compensated and the echoes equalized electronically by swept gain or time gain compensation (TGC). As soon as the transducer is pulsed, the decibel gain of the amplifier is steadily and automatically increased, in proportion to the time that has elapsed and the distance that has been traveled by the sound. In this way, all echoes from identical interfaces are rendered the same, independent of their depth, as seen in Fig. 7.12c.

Swept gain is typically varied from 0 to 50 dB. Figure 7.12d plots the applied gain in decibels against depth in tissue. To make best use of the available TGC in the region of greatest interest (and not waste it while the beam is traveling through, for example, a filled bladder) the decibel gain is not usually applied until the region of interest is reached at the threshold depth T_1. It is then increased linearly through the region of interest until depth T_2. The threshold and the slope of the ramp can be varied by the operator, and the resulting TGC curve (Fig. 7.12d) can be displayed on the screen.

7.7 B-MODE (BRIGHTNESS MODE IMAGING)

In B-mode a slice through the patient is imaged. The transducer is pulsed at regular intervals, as in A-mode, but, unlike A-mode:

◆ The ultrasound pencil beam scans back and forth across a two-dimensional section of the patient in either a linear, rectangular (Fig. 7.13a) or a sector (Fig. 7.13b) pattern. The diagram shows the scan lines traveled by each pulse of ultrasound which make up the image. Only boundaries approximately perpendicular to the scan lines will be imaged.

◆ Each time the transducer is energized, the ultrasound beam takes a new 'scan line' through the patient, and the trace starts at a point on the monitor screen corresponding to the skin surface and travels in the same direction as the ultrasound ray (Fig. 7.13c).

◆ The trace itself is suppressed.

◆ The returning echo pulses are displayed not as 'blips' but as small bright dots corresponding to each of the interfaces encountered by each ray. Figure 7.13c shows the appearance on the screen. TGC is used, as described above.

7.8 REAL-TIME IMAGING

In modern B-scanners, the image is automatically scanned in a succession of 'frames' sufficiently rapidly to demonstrate the motion of tissues.

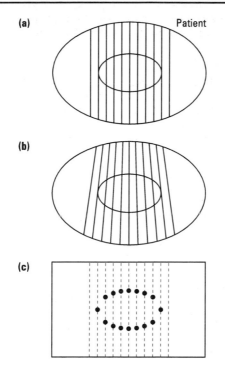

(a) Patient

(b)

(c)

Fig. 7.13 B-mode: (a) linear scan, (b) sector scan, and (c) the monitor screen.

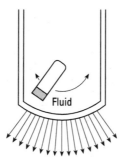

Fluid

Fig. 7.14 Mechanical sector scanner with an oscillating transducer.

Real-time imaging also allows a rapid search through a large organ. There are several methods.

Mechanical (sector) scanning

The transducer, which is a circular disk and may be an annular array, moves within a fluid-filled plastic dome pressed against the body.

In one design, illustrated in Fig. 7.14, the transducer is oscillated by an electric motor. (Alternatively, the transducer may be fixed and the sound

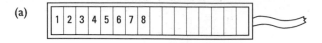

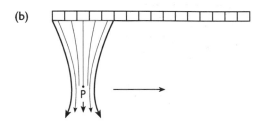

Fig. 7.15 Linear transducer array. (a) Transducer face. (b) Cross section through transducer and ultrasound beam.

reflected by an oscillating mirror.) It has the advantage that the wobble or sector angle, and so the field size, can be varied.

In another design, 3–5 transducers are mounted on a rotating wheel. Only the transducer nearest to the patient at any time is energized.

In either case, the ultrasonic beam sweeps across a sector of the body; each sweep produces one image frame. The rate of oscillation or rotation, and so the frame rate, can be varied.

Electronic scanning: stepped linear array

An elongated transducer, say 10×100 mm (shown in plan and section in Fig. 7.15) is divided into a large number (128 or more) of separate narrow strips, each about a wavelength in width. Individually they would each give a poor beam, with a short near field and widely diverging far field. The piezoelectric elements are therefore energized in overlapping groups, in succession – say, 1–6, 2–7, 3–8, ... – so that a well-defined ultrasound beam comes in effect from a small (square) transducer and scans a rectangular area in the body with (say) 120 scan lines.

Electronic focusing. In fact, however, the outermost pair of strips in each group are energized first, then after a very short delay the next pair, and finally the innermost pair, so that pulses all arrive at some point (P) at the same time, and reinforce. Figure 7.15 shows the beam shape; it is focused in the region of P. The timing of the applied pulses can be varied in order to change the focal depth P.

Electronic sector scanner: steered or phased array

The similar but shorter transducer (shown in plan and section in Fig. 7.16) contains fewer elements. If they are energized simultaneously they act as a single transducer, and the beam travels forward. If they are energized separately in rapid sequence 1, 2, 3, ..., the pulses reinforce only in one direction. They interfere destructively in all others, and the beam swings to the right. If they are energized in the reverse sequence, ..., 3, 2, 1, the beam swings to the left. By slightly changing the time delay sequence between

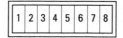

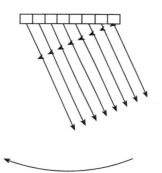

Fig. 7.16 Steered beam produced by a phased array. (a) Transducer face. (b) Cross section through transducer and ultrasound beam.

each pulse, the scan line is swept across the patient, covering a sector field (as with mechanical sector scanning).

Figure 7.16 does not show how, as with the linear array, the beam is in addition focused electronically at a selected depth by an adjustment to the phase delay pattern.

Focal depth

With both types of array, the focal length can be altered electronically by the operator: the greater the time delays between the energization of the successive pairs of elements, the shorter the focal length. Unlike the circular annular array, the beam is focused electronically in one plane only, the 'azimuthal' plane. Focusing in the other plane is done by an acoustic lens, and this defines the slice thickness.

Focusing of the beam improves the image in the focal region but makes it worse beyond it. This can be mitigated by *multiple-zone focusing*. Along each scan line, three (or four) pulses are sent in succession at the usual PRF. Each time, the phase delays are altered to focus at a different depth, both for transmission and reception. Each time, the transducer is gated so that it receives echoes from the corresponding focal zone only. Echoes arriving earlier from nearer points or later from deeper points are blocked. The focal zones overlap slightly so that the image shows no joins. Three (or four) times fewer frames can be scanned each second.

Aspects of real-time imaging

Scan line density. The patient's tissues are in effect 'sampled' along a number of scan lines or 'lines of sight', depending on the number of elements in a multielement array. To obtain good quality images with high resolution, each frame must be made up of a sufficiently large number of scan lines. In fact, about 100 lines/frame suffice because the lateral resolution is in any case limited (see Section 7.10).

Frame rate.   To follow moving tissues, a sufficiently large number of frames must be scanned each second. The frame repetition frequency depends on the number of lines per frame, and is increased by increasing the PRF:

$$\text{frame rate} \times \text{lines per frame} = \text{PRF}$$

To take a typical example, 30 frames s^{-1} each of 100 lines/frame require a PRF of 3 kHz.

Depth of view.   To image structures at depth, each pulse must have time to make the return journey from the deepest tissue before the next pulse is generated. The depth of view is increased by reducing the PRF:

$$\text{depth of view} = \frac{0.5 \times \text{sound velocity}}{\text{PRF}}$$

It is therefore not possible to achieve both a high frame rate (frame repetition frequency) and a high scan line density and at the same time produce an image with a large depth of view. One or more aspects have to be compromised.

Combining the above equations:

$$\text{Depth of view} \times (\text{scan lines/view}) \times (\text{frame rate}) = \text{constant}$$

For example, a depth of 20 cm allows 30 frames s^{-1} and 100 lines/frame.

Sector scan versus linear scan

A linear scan needs a larger area of access; gives a better quality image; maintains a wide field of view near the skin; and is used in imaging the whole abdomen, liver, superficial vessels, and thyroid, and is also used in gynaecology.

A sector scan is easier to manipulate; requires a smaller acoustic window; has a narrower field near the skin but a wider field at depth; is used to image the heart through intercostal spaces or subcostally; and infant brain through the fontanel. It is also used in intracavitary probes.

A linear array can be made in a curved format to produce a sector-type image without the complications of beam steering.

Sector scan: mechanical versus electronic

A mechanical scanner is cheaper; employs a circular transducer focused by a lens or annular array, giving better resolution. An electronic scanner has no moving parts and is more compact.

To avoid the obscuring effects of bone or gas, two types of scanner may be used endoscopically: a linear array or a single high-frequency transducer rotating through 360°. The heart may be imaged via the esophagus, the prostate via the rectum, and the fetus from the vagina.

7.9 GREY SCALE IMAGING

Tissue differentiation is made possible by making the brightness of each 'dot' in the image vary according to the strength of the corresponding echo. This necessitates using a computer, and the grey scale image is presented

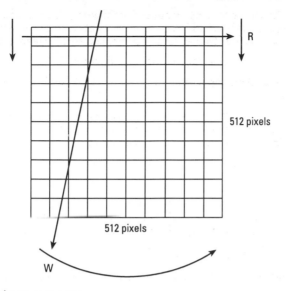

512 pixels

512 pixels

R

W

Fig. 7.17 Digital scan converter.

on the monitor screen as a matrix of (say) 512 × 512 pixels, corresponding to a similar matrix of memory locations, each 6–8 bits deep, in the core memory. Figure 7.17 can be taken to refer equally to these two matrices and to the corresponding matrix of voxels in the body.

'Write' mode

As the successive echoes arrive at the transducer, their amplitudes (after digitization) are entered, along the corresponding scan lines (such as W in Fig. 7.17), in memory locations corresponding to the voxels in the body section from which the echoes have arisen. The figures are continually updated.

For any pixel not covered by a scan line, a figure is interpolated from adjacent memory locations. The matrix 512 × 512 is greater than the number of scan lines, so that its pixel structure is not noticeable. The scan lines, however, can be obvious, especially at depth in a sector scan. They may be made less so by mathematically interpolating additional lines between those scanned.

'Read' mode

Throughout the scan and for as long as may be required thereafter, the memory locations are scanned along a series of horizontal lines (such as R in Fig. 7.17) in the form of a television raster, and the numbers read out, without destroying them. After passage through a digital-to-analog converter the signal is used to modulate the brightness of pixels on the monitor screen. Because the memory locations are written in a different order from that in which they are read, the system is called a *digital scan converter*.

The image can be retained in the computer memory while succeeding scans are carried out and stored in other 'frames'. Any frame can then be selected for display. Frame averaging can be carried out, in which 5–10 successive echoes from the same point can be stored in the same memory location, producing a time-average value. Performed pixel by pixel over the whole frame, this smooths the picture and reduces speckle.

Images can be stored in the usual ways. Hard copy can be produced from a high-resolution screen with a multiformat camera or using a laser imager. The computer is also responsible for timing and shaping the ultrasound pulse and for correlating the start and direction of each scan line on the screen with those of the corresponding sound ray.

Dynamic range

The smallest signal that can be detected is just greater than the noise, which, in ultrasound, is principally electronic noise: statistical fluctuations in the number of electrons in the very small currents. Some additional noise may be due to reverberations in the patient or in the transducer probe.

The dynamic range of any component of an ultrasound imager is the ratio of the maximum intensity of the signal to the minimum that can be detected. Taking into account the weakness of reflections from some interfaces (Table 7.3) and the attenuation of the beam, the ratio of the strongest to the weakest echoes is typically 70–80 dB. After TGC the dynamic range is typically 40–50 dB.

The monitor can display a brightness (grey scale) range of only 20 or 30 dB, within which the eye can distinguish only some 30 grey levels. It is therefore necessary to compress electronically (with a 'logarithmic amplifier') the signal amplitudes from a 40–50 dB range down to a 20–30 dB range. This may be done in such a manner as to enhance low-level, medium-level or high-level signals as required.

It is necessary to use at least an 8-bit computer which is able to store $2^8 = 256$ different echo levels, corresponding to a dynamic range of 24 dB. The dynamic range of recording film is not as good as that of the monitor, and that of Polaroid film is even worse.

7.10 RESOLUTION

Axial or depth resolution is the ability to separate two interfaces A and B along the same scan line. If, as in Fig. 7.18a, they are too close together, the echo pulses A and B will overlap and be recorded as a single interface. The axial resolution is about half the pulse length. The higher the frequency of ultrasound or the shorter the pulse, the better the axial resolution. It would be made worse by omitting the backing block and thereby increasing Q.

Lateral resolution is the ability to separate two structures side by side at the same depth. This depends on the beam width being narrower than the gap. If, as in Fig. 7.18b, the structures C and D are too close together, echoes will continue to be received as the beam, which is a few millimeters wide, sweeps across the gap between them. They will be imaged as a single structure. Resolution in the near field is improved by using a smaller transducer and by focusing.

In the case of a focused transducer, the beam is narrowest and the

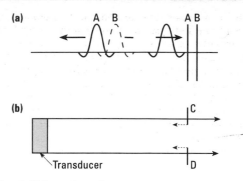

Fig. 7.18 (a) Axial and (b) lateral resolution.

resolution best in the focal region. There the *approximate beam width* = *focal length* × *wavelength / diameter*. The shorter the focal length, the narrower (and shorter) the focal region. With any particular diameter: using a higher frequency improves the resolution but reduces the penetration.

In the focal area, axial resolution may be about one wavelength and lateral resolution about three times worse, being about one-third of the transducer diameter.

Resolution and penetration

In choosing a transducer frequency for a particular investigation, it is necessary to compromise between the conflicting requirements of penetration depth (which decreases) and image resolution (which improves as the frequency is increased). Typical figures are:

3.5–5 MHz   For general-purpose abdominal scanning including heart, liver, and uterus.

5–10 MHz   For thyroid, carotid, breast, testis, and other superficial tissues, and for infants.

10–15 MHz   For the eye, which is small and acoustically transparent.

Higher frequencies still may be used in dermatology.

7.11 ARTEFACTS

Image formation assumes that sound travels in straight lines, with a constant velocity and (for TGC purposes) constant attenuation and is reflected only once from each interface; none of which hold exactly.

Speckle. Interference between the waves scattered from many small structures, too small and close to be resolved, within tissue (e.g. in liver, kidney, pancreas, and spleen) produces a textured appearance. The echo pattern is random and unrelated to the actual pattern of scatterers within the organ but it may be sufficiently characteristic to assist in tissue differentiation. On the other hand, the interiors of the bladder, cysts, large blood vessels, etc. are largely anechoic.

Reverberation. Multiple reflections to and fro between the transducer face and a relatively strongly reflecting interface near the surface (or between two such interfaces) produce a series of delayed echoes which are displayed as spurious distant structures.

Double reflection. For example, the diaphragm acts like a mirror and structures in the liver can appear to lie in the lung.

Acoustic shadowing. Strongly attenuating or reflecting structures (e.g. bowel gas, lung, bone, and gall and kidney stones) reduce the intensity of echoes from the region behind them, and cast shadows.

Acoustic enhancement. Fluid-filled structures (e.g. a cyst or a filled bladder), being weakly attenuating, increase the intensity of echoes from the region behind them, producing a 'negative shadow'. Acoustic shadowing and enhancement are made worse by TGC.

Refraction. Refraction of a beam falling obliquely on the two surfaces of bone (e.g. the skull) displaces the beam and the images of structures beyond. It distorts the image. So do variations of velocity, sound traveling significantly faster than the assumed 1540 m s^{-1} in some tissues (e.g. gall stones), and more slowly in others (e.g. lung).

7.12 M-MODE (TIME–MOTION)

The heart valves and heart wall move too quickly to be followed with a normal real-time scanner. Instead, a B-mode image is frozen on the screen and used to direct the beam from a stationary transducer (as in A-mode) along a line of interest, intersecting the moving surfaces of the heart as nearly as possible at right angles (a, b, c, d in Fig. 7.19a). Echoes are displayed on the screen (Fig. 7.19b) as a line of (moving) bright dots, as in B-mode. Movement of the heart valves along the line of sight may be displayed by stepping the vertical line of dots slowly and steadily in a horizontal direction across the screen. It may be recorded from a stationary trace on moving ultraviolet recording paper.

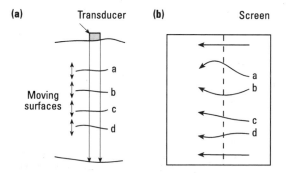

Fig. 7.19 M-mode. (a) Section through transducer and patient. (b) Appearance on monitor screen.

7.13 DOPPLER METHODS

Doppler effect

The Doppler effect is familiar to those who have heard a siren sounding on an emergency vehicle as it passes by. When (Fig. 7.20) sound waves I of frequency f are reflected at right angles, by a moving interface which is approaching the transducer, the waves are compressed. The wavelength is reduced, and (the velocity being constant) the frequency f' of the reflected wave R is increased. With a receding reflector, the frequency is reduced.

The *change* of frequency is proportional to the velocity of the interface.

$$\frac{\text{change of frequency}}{\text{original frequency}} = 2 \times \frac{\text{velocity of the interface}}{\text{velocity of sound}}$$

The higher the transducer frequency or the faster the interface moves, the greater the Doppler frequency shift. For example, if the velocity of the interface $v = 30$ cm s^{-1}, and the frequency of the transducer $f = 10$ MHz, since the velocity of sound $c = 1540$ m s^{-1} then the change of frequency $f - f'$ ≈ 4 kHz. The Doppler frequency $(f - f')$ is comparatively small and equivalent to an audio frequency, 0–10 kHz.

The above example refers to motion in the direction of the sound; motion at right angles to the transducer shows no Doppler effect and that at an angle θ has a reduced effect:

$$(f - f')f = 2(v/c) \cos \theta$$

(for the meaning of θ, sometimes called the 'angle of insonation', see Fig. 7.21). The maximum Doppler shift is obtained when $\theta = 0°$, whereas in imaging the strongest echoes occur when $\theta = 90°$.

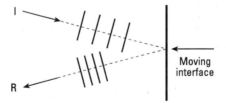

I

R

Moving interface

Fig. 7.20 Doppler effect.

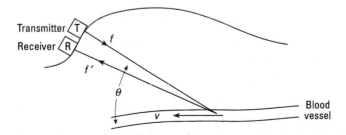

Transmitter T
Receiver R

f

f'

θ

v

Blood vessel

Fig. 7.21 Continuous-wave Doppler: detection of blood flow in a vessel.

The *change* of frequency is measured and shows how *fast* the reflector is moving toward or away from the transducer. It is also possible to detect electronically whether the frequency increases or decreases, and this shows the *direction* of movement.

7.13.1 Continuous-wave Doppler

Blood flow velocity is measured by the Doppler shift of ultrasound back scattered by the blood cells. As shown in Fig. 7.21, the probe uses two, slightly angled, transducers. They are chosen, as regards operating frequency, in the range 2–10 MHz, according to the depth of the vessel. To make the resonant frequency precise and maximize sound output, a high Q is necessary, and no backing block is used. The transmitter T is energized continuously with a radiofrequency alternating voltage of frequency f. The receiver R listens continuously to the back-scattered waves of frequency f' coming from the crossover area or 'sensitive volume'.

The original frequency f is suppressed and a Doppler signal, having the difference (or 'beat') frequency $(f - f')$, is extracted electronically. Pulsatile flow involves a range of velocities and produces a spectrum of Doppler frequencies which can be displayed on the screen, using a frequency analyzer in the manner described below.

The Doppler beat signal can be heard through a loudspeaker or headphones as a rushing sound – an audible indication of the spread of velocities involved in a heart beat. The higher the pitch the greater the velocity; the harsher the sound the greater the turbulence. An audible signal is a useful adjunct to Doppler imaging. It also forms the basis of the ultrasonic stethoscope, used to monitor the fetal heartbeat.

With a continuous wave it is not possible to locate the moving reflector or to distinguish between the flow in two overlapping vessels at different depths in the beam. On the other hand, with the short pulses used in imaging, it is not possible to get accurate Doppler flow information. A compromise using longer pulses allows some information to be obtained about both flow and location.

7.13.2 Pulsed Doppler: range gating

In *duplex* scanning, Doppler measurement is combined with a real time B-scan image. In the simplest case, the scanning head combines a single pulsed Doppler transducer offset to a mechanical or electronic sector scanner. Most of the time is spent in the Doppler mode, the B-scan image being updated once a second. The imaging frequency is chosen to optimize resolution. The Doppler transducer might operate at a lower frequency, which, as described below, allows faster flow to be measured.

A real-time B-mode image is produced, and with its help a line of sight is chosen for the Doppler beam. Along it, cursors are set to identify the *sampling volume* (A in Fig. 7.23a) which is positioned over the vessel in which blood flow is to be measured. If the vessel is clearly defined, the angle θ can be read off, to allow measured frequency shifts to be converted into blood flow velocities. The diameter of the lumen of the vessel can also be estimated, to allow volume flow rates to be calculated, at least approximately.

The normal short imaging pulses are interspersed with bursts of 'Doppler' ultrasound, each some 10 cycles long. A '*range gate*' is set to accept only those echoes which arrive within a short interval at a specific time, so that they can have come only from the selected sampling volume. The depth of the tissue so 'interrogated' depends on the time at which the gate is opened, and its thickness on the time for which it is open. The width of the sampling volume (or 'gated Doppler acquisition area'), which in practice is 'pear shaped', is the width of the Doppler beam.

Since ultrasound takes 7 μs to travel 1 cm in average soft tissue, if the gate is opened 70 μs after the transducer is pulsed and closed 7 μs later, blood velocities will be sampled in tissue about 5 mm thick at a depth of 5 cm.

The intervals between pulses must be long enough for the successive Doppler signals not to overlap. A high PRF is chosen for superficial vessels, and a lower one for deeper vessels. As the range setting is increased, the PRF is reduced and the TGC automatically increased.

The Doppler signal comprises a wide range of audio frequencies corresponding to the range of blood velocities in the sampling volume. It can be analyzed and displayed as a time–velocity spectrum or sonogram. An electrocardiogram trace can be displayed at the same time.

Sonogram

A sonogram is a graph of Doppler frequency against time, and displays the variation of blood flow velocity and direction during the heart cycle. It is bounded by an upper curve showing the variation of maximum flow velocity and a lower curve showing that of minimum flow velocity. As sketched in Fig. 7.22, the area between the curves is filled with 'pixels', each in practice say 10 ms wide and 100 Hz tall.

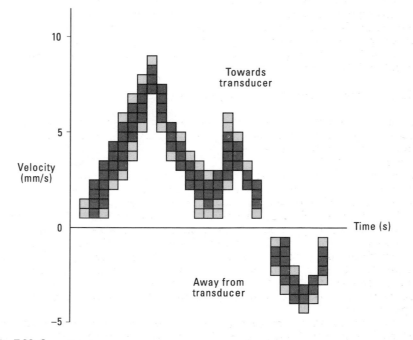

Fig. 7.22 Sonogram.

The Doppler signal is continuously sampled in a series of 10 ms 'snapshots', during each of which it is analyzed into its component frequencies and the spectrum represented as a column of pixels. Each pixel corresponds to a different frequency or flow velocity. Each pixel has a grey level representing the number of red blood cells in the sampling volume that have that velocity at that instant of time. From the sonogram, parameters such as peak velocity, mean velocity, and variance of velocity can be evaluated.

Pressure measurement

Pressures in a stenosed artery or in the jet of blood issuing from a diseased heart valve can be estimated by Doppler measurement of flow velocity. When blood flows through a constriction, the flow velocity increases (to V m s^{-1}, say) and there is a corresponding increase in pressure (P mmHg) given by the modified Bernouiili formula $P = 4V^2$. This formula is a simplification of the Bernouilli equation which expresses the facts that blood is incompressible and that energy is conserved but ignores any effects of viscosity and turbulence.

Aliasing

With pulsed Doppler it is not possible to measure very high-flow velocities with accuracy. If the flow is too fast it will be shown in the wrong direction and its velocity underestimated. This artefact shows as 'wrap-round' top and bottom in the sonogram, and is known as 'aliaising'.

The same artefact can be seen in the cinema when the spoked wheel of a stagecoach rotates so fast that it appears to turn backwards, as described in Section 9.2. Aliasing is a consequence of the sampling requirement (associated with the names of Shannon and Nyquist) that *the waveform being measured (i.e. the Doppler signal) must be 'sampled' at least twice in each period*.

In other words, the frequency with which the Doppler pulses are repeated must be at least twice the maximum Doppler shift frequency produced by the flow. Thus the fastest flow that can be measured with accuracy is the velocity which produces a Doppler shift frequency equal to half the PRF being used. A greater flow velocity than this produces 'aliasing'. Aliasing does not occur with continuous-wave Doppler.

It is therefore particularly difficult to measure fast flow in deep blood vessels. The deeper the gate has to be set, the smaller the PRF that can be used (see Section 7.8), and so the smaller the fastest flow that can be measured without aliasing.

For example, if the Doppler shift frequency produced by the fast blood flow associated with a stenosis is 8 kHz, the PRF must be at least 16 kHz. This allows a listening time of only 60 μs between pulses, in which time the sound can travel to and fro through a depth of view of only 5 cm.

The depth of the sampling volume determines the PRF needed, and the PRF determines the maximum velocity that can be measured without aliasing. Thus:

maximum velocity (cm s^{-1}) × range (cm) × transducer frequency (MHz) ≈ 4000

The risk of aliasing can be reduced by reducing the Doppler effect by (a) using a probe of lower frequency f or (b) increasing the angle θ; but both

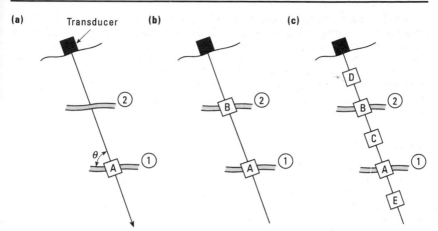

Fig. 7.23 Pulsed Doppler (a) normal and (b, c) high PRF modes ① and ② are blood vessels.

increase the error in the measured flow. The risk can also be reduced by (c) increasing the PRF, but this causes problems, as we shall now see.

High pulse repetition frequency mode

Suppose that the gate is set to measure the blood velocity in the selected sample volume A (Fig. 7.23a). Normally the PRF would be set so that there is just time to collect the Doppler echo from A before the transducer is pulsed again. This means that it is not possible to measure the flow velocity if it is very high. This can partially be overcome by the use of a 'high PRF' mode.

Suppose that the PRF is doubled; this will double the maximum measurable blood flow velocity. Unfortunately, at the moment when a Doppler echo from A is being accepted, so is one produced by the next pulse, coming from a sample volume B at exactly half the depth of A (Fig. 7.23b). Sonograms from the two samples would be superimposed on the display. The operator must therefore position the beam in such a way that only sample volume A is placed on a vessel while the nearer sample volume B is placed over an area of little perfusion.

Quadrupling the PRF will further improve the measurement of velocity. It does so at the expense of superimposing velocity data from multiple gated volumes (A, B, C, D and E in Fig. 7.23c). Ambiguity in velocity has been replaced by ambiguity in range. Carrying the idea to the extreme, when the PRF becomes very high, the pulses merge, and we have reinvented continuous-wave Doppler with no aliasing but no range data.

7.13.3 Real-time color flow imaging

Whereas a grey scale (B-mode) image shows the strength of echo coming from each pixel, a *color-mapped Doppler* image shows the direction and velocity of movement or flow occurring in each pixel by means of an arbitrary color code, e.g.

Flow toward the transducer: red
Flow away from the transducer: blue
Turbulence (i.e. variations in flow direction): green or yellow

The depth of each color varies with the velocity of flow, stationary tissues appearing grey.

A real time B-mode scanner is used, and the Doppler color overlay switched on and off at will. Compared with normal B-scan imaging, the Doppler pulse is longer, being a compromise between accurate depth information requiring a short pulse and accurate velocity information requiring a longer pulse. To obtain the latter, a number of Doppler pulses have to be sent in succession along each scan line.

Typically, 25 frames are scanned a second over a 60° sector. In each frame, the beam is steered in succession along 64 scan lines, dwelling on each line long enough for a B-scan pulse followed by a train of, say, eight consecutive Doppler pulses to be sent in and the echoes to return. Along each line the Doppler echoes from 128 separate gated ranges, each 1.5 mm long, are collected and analyzed for frequency. The *average velocity* is evaluated in each sample volume, about 3 mm in size, and represented by the depth of color of the corresponding pixel.

Whereas the sonogram in a gated Doppler image is produced from, say, 100 consecutive pulses (and effectively from an infinite number in continuous-wave Doppler), in color scanning there is time to send only some 4–12 pulses along each scan line. The data acquired are sufficient only to estimate the mean velocity and variance of velocity (as a measure of turbulence) in each sample volume and to color each pixel accordingly.

To produce the sonogram of any sample volume or to measure peak velocity, a single sample volume is selected on the color scan and the instrument switched to spectral Doppler mode.

The performance of color scan Doppler is limited by the small time available to collect the data from each beam position. The following factors can be varied, and are interrelated:

- *frame rate*, which should be fast enough to follow changes of flow velocity;
- *penetration depth*, which is inversely proportional to PRF;
- *field width* or sector size (30–90°)
- *line density*, i.e. scan lines per frame, which should be high enough for good spatial resolution;
- *number of pulses in a train*, which should be high enough to give accurate velocity information.

Increasing any one of the above entails reducing one or more of the others. The sector size and depth range should be set as small as possible, especially with children, where a high frame rate is desirable.

To achieve the required number of scan lines and the required frame rate, it may be necessary to restrict color mapping to a selected part of the B-scan grey scale image.

Aliasing

Aliasing is also a feature of color scans since the PRF has to be set low enough to accommodate the deepest sampling volume in the image. Blue becomes red, and vice versa. High-velocity laminar flow appears with an aliased blue center and a nonaliased red edge. High-speed jets with associated turbulence show up as a colored mosaic. Having located such high-velocity features, the machine can be switched to continuous-wave or pulsed Doppler for more accurate measurement and sonogram display.

7.14 SAFETY CONSIDERATIONS

Ultrasound is not an electromagnetic radiation, and is nonionizing. It is a low-risk as well as a low-cost method of medical imaging.

The intensity of an ultrasound beam is greatest in the focal region, where it is typically 0.1 mW mm^{-2}, averaged over the examination. The peak intensity (during the brief pulse) is likely to be 1000-fold greater.

There has been no confirmed evidence of damage from diagnostic ultrasound exposure. The output of each probe should be checked periodically, and operators should keep within the agreed safety guidelines:

- the time-averaged intensity should nowhere exceed 100 mW cm^{-2};
- the total sound energy (intensity × dwell time) should nowhere exceed 50 J cm^{-2}.

Imaging systems rarely approach these levels, but pulsed Doppler systems often do, and should be used with caution.

If either of the above figures were grossly exceeded there would be risk from:

- Local *heating*, due to frictional, viscous, and molecular relaxation processes, leading to chemical damage, but mitigated by bloodflow. (This heating effect is used therapeutically.)
- Acoustic *streaming* of cellular contents in the direction of the beam, affecting cell membrane permeability
- *Cavitation*: the high peak pressure changes causing microbubbles in a liquid or near-liquid medium to expand. If they did so to the point of very sudden collapse there might be an enormous rise of temperature with consequent profound chemical damage to cellular constituents. This is less likely to occur with pulsed beams as each pulse does not last long enough for resonance to be reached.
- *Mechanical damage* to cell membranes due to violent acceleration of particles.

7.15 QUALITY ASSURANCE

- Resolution is tested by imaging a test rig composed of parallel wires mounted on a frame and immersed in a Perspex bath containing a fluid in which sound travels at 1540 m s^{-1}.
- Another test involves imaging a Perspex block. A number of equally spaced images of decreasing brightness are obtained corresponding to multiple reflections. This can be used to monitor (a) sensitivity, (b) dynamic range, and (c) accuracy of the A-scan caliper. Since sound travels faster in Perspex than tissue, each 7 mm of Perspex is equivalent to 4 mm of tissue.
- More complicated test objects are required to assess grey scale performance and Doppler function.

◆ The power output of the transducer is measured by 'weighing' the sound pressure with a force balance or by measuring the heating effect using a calorimeter. More sophisticated techniques can be used to measure the intensity distribution (beam shape).

7.16 APPENDIX

Decibel notation. A wide range of power or intensity ratios can be compressed by using a logarithmic scale as follows:

$$10 \times \log (\text{power or intensity ratio}) = \text{No. of decibels (dB)}$$

For example

Ratio:	1000/1	100/1	20/1	10/1	2/1	1/1	1/2	1/10	1/100
dB:	30	20	13	10	3	0	-3	-10	-20

Note that decibel values are additive. Positive values show amplification and negative values attenuation.

VIVA QUESTIONS

1. What is the definition of ultrasound?
2. What is the relationship between velocity, wavelength, and frequency?
3. What is meant by 'impedance'?
4. What is a piezoelectric material and how does it work?
5. How may a transducer be focused?
6. Draw a diagram of the sound beam for a single-focus transducer.
7. What types of transducer are used for real-time scanners? Compare and contrast them.
8. What is the Doppler effect in ultrasound and how does a Doppler ultrasound system work?
9. Explain the differences between continuous, pulsed, and color Doppler modalities used in ultrasound diagnosis.
10. What do the terms 'acoustic shadowing', 'acoustic enhancement', and 'reverberation' mean?
11. Name three causes of artefacts in ultrasound and explain them.
12. What is the velocity of ultrasound in tissues? Is it the same for all tissues? How does it compare with other materials?
13. Why cannot tissues behind air-filled structures or bone be seen?
14. What are the hazards of ultrasound?

MAGNETIC RESONANCE IMAGING

Magnetic resonance imaging (MRI) employs radiowaves and magnetic fields. The patient is placed in a magnet, and a radiowave sent in. The transmitter is turned off, and the patient re-emits radiowaves, which are received and used for reconstruction of the image. It is the nuclei of hydrogen atoms in water (free or attached to other molecules) and fat which absorb and emit the radiofrequency (RF) energy.

MRI is able to measure the hydrogen content, in a particularly subtle way, of individual voxels in a slice of the patient and represent it as a shade of grey in the corresponding pixel on the screen.

Although the nuclei of all atoms contain protons and many nuclides possess the property called nuclear magnetic resonance, we shall (until Section 8.9) consider only hydrogen and use the term 'proton' to refer only to the hydrogen nucleus.

8.1 THE SPINNING PROTON

A proton spins continually like a top around an axis called the spin vector. The circulating charge is like a small loop of current, and each proton acts like a bar magnet or dipole. Its magnetic moment m is represented by a vector joining the north and south poles, drawn as an arrow in Fig. 8.1. Normally, all the individual dipoles point in a random fashion, with equal numbers in every direction. The net magnetic effect is then zero. (This ignores the tiny effect upon them of the earth's magnetic field.)

The patient lies prone or supine in a solenoid coil (the outermost coil in Fig. 8.2) carrying a direct current (DC). This produces everywhere inside the coil a very uniform and strong magnetic field, represented by a vector B pointing along the axis of the coil. This is taken as the Z-axis; the Y-axis

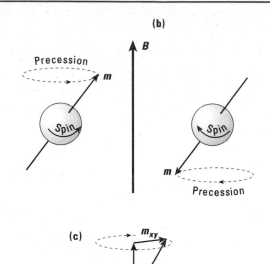

Fig. 8.1 The magnetic vectors associated with a spinning proton precessing (a) parallel and (b) antiparallel to a magnetic field. (c) The transverse and longitudinal components of the magnetic vector.

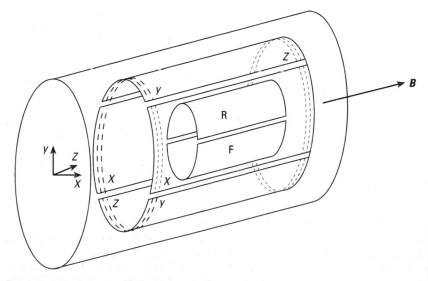

Fig. 8.2 Arrangement of the coils in an MR machine.

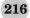

runs vertically from top to bottom, and the X-axis horizontally across the machine. The magnetic field strength has a set value between 0.15–2.0 tesla (T), depending on the machine. By way of example, throughout this chapter we will take a machine with a field strength of 1 T. This is some 20 000 times greater than the earth's magnetic field.

Inside the coil, the patient becomes very slightly magnetized. The static magnetic field B causes the magnetic dipoles to turn and point along the Z-axis in one of two stable directions – either, as in Fig. 8.1a, in the direction of the field (parallel or 'spin-up') or, as in Fig. 8.1b, in the opposite direction (antiparallel or 'spin down').

Due to thermal jostling, the state which needs less energy is preferred. Very slightly more dipoles point spin up than spin down. MRI depends on detecting this small difference, which is proportional to B and amounts to about 3 out of each million protons at 1 T.

Most of the dipoles, each with a magnetic moment m, cancel each other out in pairs (parallel and antiparallel), and those not so paired produce a combined, longitudinal net or bulk magnetic vector M_z in the direction of B.

Henceforth the terms 'spins' or 'protons' will refer only to the *detectable* protons, the excess of spin-up over spin-down protons, and we will ignore the others. For example, in a cubic millimeter of water there are about 7×10^{19} protons, of which only some 2×10^{14} will be detectable.

Precession

The static field also causes the spinning protons to 'wobble' in a regular manner called precession (Fig. 8.1a,b). The direction of the spin axis tilts and rotates around the direction of the magnetic field B with a fixed frequency (millions of revolutions per second), called the Larmor frequency. Figure 8.1 makes clear the difference between spin, precession, and the magnetic moment m of a single proton.

This is similar to the way in which the north–south axis of the earth precesses once in 25 000 years, due to the gravitational pull of the sun, and a spinning top or gyroscope precesses, due to the earth's gravitational field.

The tilting of the spin axis of a precessing proton splits its magnetic vector m into a longitudinal component m_z which points in the Z-direction, and a transverse component m_{xy} which rotates in the XY plane (Fig. 8.1c).

Now consider all the detectable protons in a single voxel of tissue (size a few cubic millimeters, illustrated in Fig. 8.3). The m_z vectors all point in the Z-direction and add up to a combined or net longitudinal magnetism M_z (Fig. 8.3a). This cannot be measured directly as it points in the same direction as B. Because the protons precess independently their m_{xy} vectors point in all directions and cancel out. The net transverse magnetism $M_{xy} = 0$.

The stronger the magnetic field, the faster a proton precesses. The frequency of precession (f) or Larmor frequency is proportional to the product of:

◆ the magnetic field strength: and
◆ a property of the nucleus called the gyromagnetic ratio γ.

For example, for hydrogen nuclei in a field of 1 T, $f = 42.6$ MHz. This is an RF, and has a very precise value (in water, within ±0.1 Hz).

In the quantum theory, a frequency of 42.6 MHz corresponds to a quantum energy of 0.2 μeV. The energy of the antiparallel state is therefore 0.2 μeV

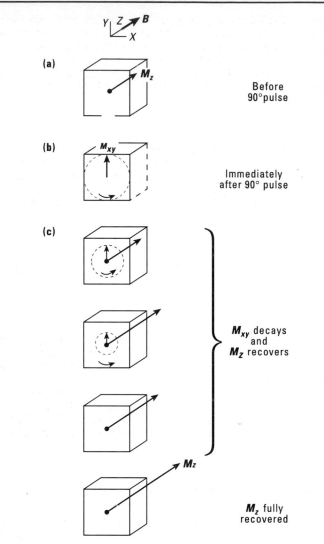

Fig. 8.3 The net magnetization in a voxel: a time sequence following a 90° pulse.

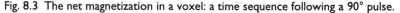

greater than that of the parallel state. It is because of this small energy difference that slightly more spins line up parallel rather than antiparallel.

Radiofrequency coils

Surrounding and close to the patient are a set of coils (the innermost coils in Fig. 8.2) connected to an RF generator (transmitter or oscillator) which sends through them a pulse of RF current lasting 1 ms or less. This produces a rapidly alternating magnetic field, in a direction perpendicular to B, which has two effects:

◆ some or all of the spin-up protons pick up energy, turn spin down, and are said to be excited. This affects M_z; it may be reduced, disappear, or even reverse, depending on the length and strength of the RF pulse.

◆ the protons are pulled into synchronism, and they now precess in step or in phase (see Section 1.10). Their m_{xy} vectors add up to a transverse magnetic vector M_{xy} which rotates in the XY plane (Fig. 8.3b) at the Larmor frequency.

Resonance

It is well known that an opera singer must strike precisely the right note to shatter a wineglass. Similarly, in order to affect the dipoles, the frequency of the RF generator must very accurately match the Larmor precession or 'resonant' frequency of the dipoles. In other words, the photon energy of the radiowaves must be exactly the same as the energy difference between spin-up and spin-down protons.

180° pulse

An RF pulse of a certain total energy will give to each and every dipole exactly the energy (0.2 μeV) required to tip them through 180°. This temporarily reverses the net magnetic vector M_z.

90° pulse

An RF pulse of half that total energy (i.e. half the intensity or half the duration) will tip half of the dipoles, so that equal numbers point spin up and spin down, thus reducing M_z to zero. The RF pulse also causes them to move into the same phase and precess together.

Together they produce a transverse magnetism M_{xy}, perpendicular to B, which rotates in the XY plane at the Larmor frequency (Fig. 8.3b). It is as if the '90° pulse' has tipped the magnetic vector M_z through 90°. MRI involves sending a series of many such 90° pulses, repeated at intervals of TR seconds, called the repetition time.

8.2 THE MAGNETIC RESONANCE SIGNAL

When the 90° pulse is over, the magnetic vector M_{xy} continues for a while to rotate in the transverse XY plane. Just like the rotating magnet in a dynamo, it induces in the RF coil an alternating (RF) voltage of a few microvolts. After amplification by an RF amplifier (receiver), tuned like a radio to the resonant frequency, the amplitude or envelope of this signal is sampled and digitized in the usual way. After processing by a computer it is used to control the pixel grey level in the MR image.

Using methods of 'spatial encoding', described in Section 8.4, the MR signal from each individual voxel in a 256 × 256 matrix can be identified.

Note that only M_{xy} produces an MR signal; M_z does not. But since M_{xy} is produced by tipping M_z, *the signal produced by a 90° pulse depends on the value of M_z immediately before that pulse is applied.*

The peak signal is proportional to and the pixel brightness depends on:

◆ proton or spin density (PD, number of protons per cubic millimeter) of the voxel;

- the gyromagnetic ratio of the nucleus; and
- the static field strength B, because placing the patient in a stronger magnetic field increases the preponderance of protons which are initially spin up over those that are spin down.

Only mobile protons give signals; those in large molecules or effectively immobilized in bone do not. The greater part of the signal is due to body water, whether free or bound to molecules. Air, in sinuses for example, having no hydrogen, produces no signal, and always appears black in the image. Fat has a higher proton density than other soft tissues. Grey matter has a somewhat greater proton density than white matter. Tissues do not, however, vary greatly in their proton densities.

Free induction decay

The MR signal is greatest immediately after the brief 90° pulse has been switched off. Thereafter the dipoles return, some earlier than others, to their original orientation and, as indicated in Fig. 8.3c, M_z regrows or 'recovers' while M_{xy} decreases or 'decays', and, accordingly, the strength of the MR signal decays, although its frequency remains the same.

At any instant of time, M_z and M_{xy} combine to produce a *sum* vector M. The 90° pulse has tipped the sum vector through 90°. Then, during relaxation, as M_z increases and M_{xy} decreases, the sum vector spirals (beehive fashion, Fig. 8.4) back from the transverse plane to the longitudinal direction. This is due to two concurrent and quite independent methods of energy loss or 'relaxation': spin–lattice and spin–spin relaxation.

Spin–lattice or T_1 relaxation

The dipoles are jostled by the thermal motion of the rest of the molecule or nearby molecules. The excited protons give up energy to the molecular 'lattice'. One by one the dipoles tip back parallel to the Z-axis, and M_z slowly reappears (Fig. 8.3). This is also called 'longitudinal relaxation'.

In Fig. 8.5 the left-hand axis refers to curve a, which shows how, after M_z has been destroyed at time 0 by the first 90° pulse, it increases again relatively slowly and does so exponentially with a time constant T_1.

T_1 is the time for M_z to recover to 63% of its maximum value. T_1 has a value of so many hundreds of milliseconds (Table 8.1). After three time constants, recovery is 95% complete:

Time:	0 ·	T_1	$2T_1$	$3T_1$
Recovery:	0	63%	87%	95%

Causes of spin–lattice relaxation

- Slow jostling by heavy molecules, being near to the resonant frequency, is most effective at removing energy from excited dipoles. Water bound to the surface of proteins has a relatively short T_1, as do the protons in fat. If a weaker magnetic field B is used, the protons precess faster, and T_1 of tissue shortens, and M_z reappears more quickly.
- Rapid jostling by light-weight molecules is relatively ineffective at removing energy from the excited dipoles. Free water, urine, amniotic fluid, cerebrospinal fluid (CSF), and other solutions of salts have a long T_1. The greater the proportion of free water in tissue, the longer is T_1.

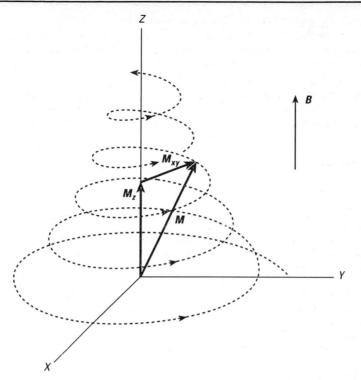

Fig. 8.4 Behavior of the sum magnetic vector **M** during free induction decay.

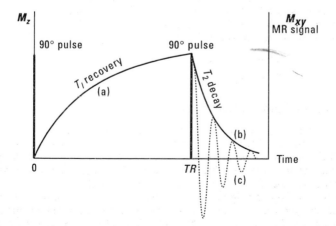

Fig. 8.5 T_1 recovery of **M**$_z$ and T_2 decay of **M**$_{xy}$.

Table 8.1 Typical relaxation times of tissues in a field of 1 T

Material	T_1 (ms)	T_2 (ms)
Fat	250	80
Liver	400	40
Kidney	550	60
Spleen	400	60
White matter	650	90
Grey matter	800	100
CSF	2000	150
Water	3000	3000
Ice	Very long	Very short

The atoms in solids and rigid macromolecules are relatively fixed and they are the least effective at removing energy. Compact bone, teeth, calculi, and metallic clips have a very long T_1.

Spin–spin or T_2 relaxation

M_z has partially recovered when, TR seconds after the first, a second 90° pulse converts the available M_z into M_{xy}. In Fig. 8.5 the right-hand axis refers to curve b, which shows how M_{xy} then decays relatively rapidly, for the following reason.

Immediately after that 90° pulse the dipoles are still all precessing in phase, and their m_{xy} vectors simply add up. The large net magnetic vector M_{xy} induces a large MR signal. The dipoles then progressively dephase as some rotate faster or slower than others. As a result, the net strength of the rotating magnetic vector M_{xy} decreases, and so does the induced signal (curve c in Fig. 8.5).

Much of this dephasing effect is due to machine factors external to the patient, which will be considered in Section 8.3, but the clinically important part is related to tissue structure and is called spin–spin, 'transverse', or T_2 relaxation.

As depicted in Fig. 8.5, M_{xy} decreases or decays exponentially (curve b), and so does the induced signal (curve c), both with a time constant T_2.

T_2 is the time for the MR signal to fall to 37% of its maximum value. T_2 has a value of so many tens of milliseconds (Table 8.1). After three time constants, only 5% of it remains:

Time:	0	$1T_2$	$2T_2$	$3T_2$
Signal:	100%	37%	14%	5%

Causes of spin–spin relaxation. The dephasing occurs because a spinning proton experiences a tiny additional magnetic field (around 1 mT) produced by each neighboring proton. Individual protons are affected slightly differently, and the magnetic field B therefore varies a little from place to place and from time to time on the submicroscopic scale. So does the rate of precession; some precess faster and some slower, and energy passes from one proton to another, or 'spin to spin'.

The local variation of magnetic field is greatest in solids and rigid macromolecules in which the atoms are relatively fixed. The dipoles in compact bone, tendons, teeth, calculi, and metallic clips dephase quickly. They have a very short T_2 and do not produce a lasting signal.

The effect is least in free water, urine, amniotic fluid, CSF, and other solutions of salts. The lighter molecules are in rapid thermal motion, which smooths out the local field and results in a long T_2. Broadly speaking, the greater the proportion of free water in tissue, the longer is T_2. Spleen has a longer relaxation time than liver, and renal medulla longer than the cortex.

Water bound to the surface of proteins and other large molecules, which move more slowly, has a shorter T_2 than free water, and so does the hydrogen in fat.

Tissue characteristics

T_2 is always shorter than T_1. T_2 is more or less unaffected by, but T_1 of tissue increases with, magnetic field strength, i.e. with resonant frequency. For example:

Magnetic field (T):	0.15	0.3	0.5	1.0	1.5
T_1 of muscle (ms):	330	440	550	730	870
T_1 of fat (ms):	170	190	210	240	260

There are no *precise* values of T_1 or T_2 for specific tissues. Figures cover a wide range, and representative, rounded-off values are given in Table 8.1. Abnormal tissue tends to have a higher PD, T_1, and T_2 than normal tissue due to increased water content or vascularity.

Since T_1 and T_2 are properties of the tissues which show more variation than proton density, they are used in forming the MR image. Comparing the range of T_1 and T_2 values for soft tissues with the computed tomography (CT) numbers of corresponding tissues given in Section 4.3 shows the superior soft tissue contrast resolution of MRI compared with CT.

8.3 SPIN-ECHO SEQUENCE

In practice the MR or 'free induction decay' (FID) signal is rarely measured because it decays so very rapidly – with a time constant T_2^* of a few milliseconds, much shorter than T_2. This happens because the static field B is not perfectly uniform:

- mainly because of the magnetic field gradient (see Section 8.4) deliberately produced across the voxel and also
- because of unintentional imperfections in the engineering of the magnet, and
- because the introduction of the patient unavoidably distorts the static field (due to magnetic susceptibility, see Section 8.10)

These systemic effects unfortunately add to the effect of spin–spin interactions in the tissue in causing some dipoles to precess faster than others after a 90° pulse, with consequent dephasing.

To remove the effects associated with the static field but leave the tissue characteristic T_2 effect, a *spin echo (SE) pulse sequence* is used. Figure 8.6a depicts one cycle of this sequence, which is repeated 256 times or more in

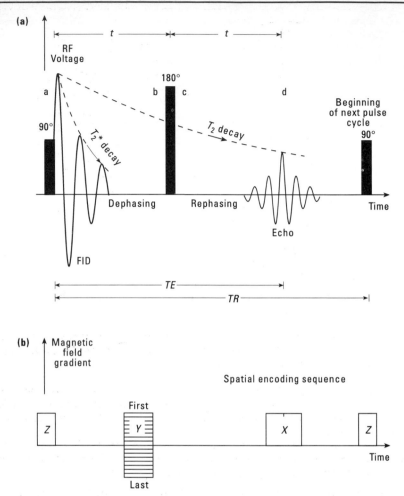

Fig. 8.6 One cycle of the SE sequence: (a) RF pulses and signal (b) magnetic field gradients.

producing one MR image frame. It should be studied in conjunction with the sequence of events (a–d) depicted in Fig. 8.7.

In the SE sequence, each 90° pulse is followed, t seconds later, by a 180° pulse. The signal is measured after a further and equal time interval (so that the 'echo time' TE = $2t$).

Step a. Immediately after the 90° pulse, the dipoles are all precessing exactly in phase (Fig. 8.7a). M_{xy} is a maximum, and so is the FID signal, but it is not measured at this stage because it decays so rapidly.

Step b. The m_{xy} vectors begin to dephase, the faster precessing ones ('leaders') getting ahead of the slower ones ('laggers' in Fig. 8.7b). M_{xy} and the FID signal decay with time constant T_2^* (extreme left, Fig. 8.6a).

Step c. After time t, the 180° pulse is applied and tips all the dipoles from spin up to spin down. This turns the individual m_{xy} vectors through 180° in

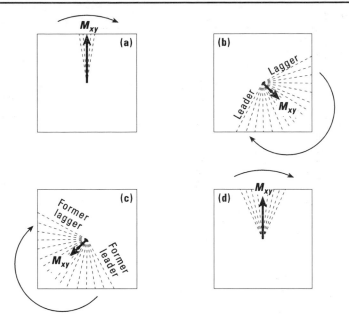

Fig. 8.7 Dephasing and rephasing of the m_{xy} vectors of individual protons in a voxel in an SE sequence: (a) immediately afer 90° pulse, (b) just before the 180° pulse, (c) just after the 180° pulse, and (d) at time TE.

the X-direction (Fig. 8.7c). Laggers become leaders, and vice versa. M_{xy} and the signal are still small. As the m_{xy} vectors continue to rotate in the XY plane they now rephase. The faster ones catch up with the slower ones, and M_{xy} and the MR signal regrow.

Step d. After a further time t they are again momentarily in phase (Fig. 8.7d), and M_{xy} and the MR signal are at their peak. Thereafter they grow out of phase again, and M_{xy} and the MR signal decay.

The 180° pulse is often called the 'rephasing' or 'refocusing' pulse. It has reversed and eliminated the dephasing effect of systemic magnetic field inhomogeneities. This leaves (Fig. 8.7d) only the residual dephasing due to the random effects of spin–spin interaction, T_2.

The MR signal reappears as an 'echo' of the initial signal (see Fig. 8.6a), and is essentially two FID signals back to back. When measured at time $TE = 2t$ it will have been reduced by T_2 relaxation. The longer is TE, the smaller the MR signal.

Tissue contrast

The MR image maps three properties (PD, T_1, and T_2) of tissue, and is controlled by two parameters set by the operator: TE or time to echo and TR or time to repeat.

The MR signal arising from a voxel and the brightness of the pixel depends on:

(a) How many protons there are in the voxel. The greater the spin density, the larger the signal and the brighter the pixel.

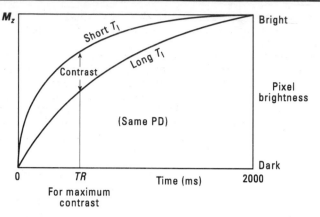

Fig. 8.8 T_1 contrast.

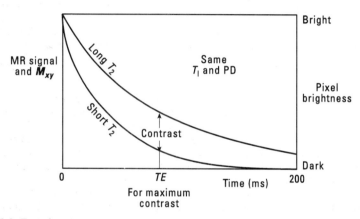

Fig. 8.9 T_2 contrast.

(b) How far M_z has recovered from the previous 90° pulse when it is tipped by the next 90° pulse, i.e. on T_1 compared to TR.

Figure 8.8 compares two tissues which differ only in T_1, their PDs being the same. It shows that the shorter T_1 or the longer TR, the greater the M_z available to be tipped and the larger the MR signal, the brighter the pixel and the better the signal-to-noise ratio.

(c) How far M_{xy} has decayed when the echo is formed, i.e. on T_2 compared to TE.

Figure 8.9 compares two tissues which differ only in T_2 (their T_1 and PD being the same). It shows that the longer T_2 or the shorter TE, the larger the MR signal, the brighter the pixel and the better the signal-to-noise ratio.

Weighted images

TE and TR are chosen so that pixel brightness depends on one of three combinations of PD, T_1, and T_2.

T₁-weighted image. Figure 8.8 shows that maximum contrast (the difference between the curves) between tissues of different T_1 is produced by a fairly short TR.

A TR of 300–800 ms is used – about the same as the average T_1 of the tissues of interest. A short TE (30 ms) is also used, as this reduces the effect of T_2 on contrast. (It cannot be much shorter as the system has to recover from the shock of the RF pulse before the MR signal can be measured.)

Image contrast is then principally due to differences in the proton density and the T_1 relaxation properties of the tissues. The shorter is T_1, the stronger the signal and the brighter the pixel. *Fat is bright*, as is fatty bone marrow, while *water and CSF are dark.*

T₂-weighted image. Figure 8.9 shows that the longer is TE, the greater the contrast between tissues of different T_2. However, it must not be so long that the signal is so small as to be obscured by background noise.

A relatively long TE of 90–140 ms is used – about the same as the average T_2 of the tissues of interest. A long TR (1000–2000 ms) is also used, as this reduces the effect of T_1, on contrast, although unfortunately it increases the imaging time.

Image contrast is then principally due to differences in the proton density and the T_2 relaxation properties of the tissues. The longer is T_2, the stronger the signal and the brighter the pixel. *Water and CSF appear brighter than fat.*

Proton density weighted image. Figure 8.10 compares two tissues which differ only in PD, their T_1 being the same. It shows that the longer is TR, the greater the contrast between tissues of different PDs.

A long TR (1000–3000 ms) is used – about $3T_1$ – and this reduces the effect of T_1 on contrast. A short as possible TE (30 ms) is used, as this reduces the effect of T_2. Generally speaking, PD weighting produces greater signal strength and less noise.

Image contrast is then principally due to differences in the proton densities of the tissues. The greater the proton density, the stronger the signal and the brighter the image. CSF, fat, and indeed most tissues, having a high proton density, appear bright.

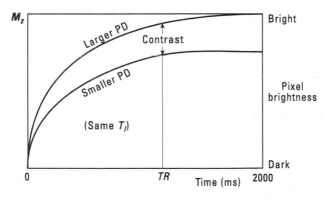

Fig. 8.10 PD contrast.

Table 8.2 T_1, T_2, and PD weighting effects

T_1-weighted	TR and TE both short	Short T_1 = bright
T_2-weighted	TE and TR both long	Long T_2 = bright
PD weighted	Short TE and long TR	High PD = bright

Summary. A large signal and a bright pixel results from tissues having a large PD and a long T_2; and from using an imager with a larger *B*. A small signal and a dark pixel results from a long T_1 and (as will be seen later) arterial blood flow. *In all images*, air and cortical bone, having no hydrogen, appear black.

TR controls the amount of T_1 weighting, and TE the amount of T_2 weighting in the image, as in Table 8.2.

In practice, matters may not be so clear cut. It is not possible to rid any image of some T_2 weighting; and relative weighting may differ from tissue to tissue across an image.

White and grey matter. In a PD-weighted image, grey matter, with its somewhat higher PD, appears brighter than white matter. In a T_2-weighted image, grey matter, with its longer T_2 and higher PD, is brighter than white matter. In a T_1-weighted image, white matter is brighter than grey matter but its shorter T_1 is somewhat counteracted by its lower PD.

The opposing effects of T_1 and T_2

T_1 and T_2 are mutually antagonistic and have opposing effects on image brightness. Generally speaking, tissues with a long T_1 also have a long T_2, and those with a short T_1 have a short T_2. This is why images cannot be weighted for both T_1 and T_2.

Remembering once again that *the signal produced by a 90° pulse depends on the value of* M_z *immediately before the pulse is applied*, Figs 8.8 and 8.9 can be combined into Fig. 8.11. It shows that, with an injudicious choice of TE and TR, tissues with quite different relaxation times can produce equal signals. Showing no contrast, they will be indistinguishable. With a shorter TE than this, the image tends to be T_1 weighted, and with a longer TE it tends to be T_2 weighted.

Other factors affecting the magnetic resonance signal and contrast

Table 8.3 shows there to be a more complex state of affairs than in X-ray imaging.

8.4 SPATIAL ENCODING

To produce an image, it is necessary to pick out the signals coming from individual voxels. This is done in three stages: slice selection, line selection, and point selection.

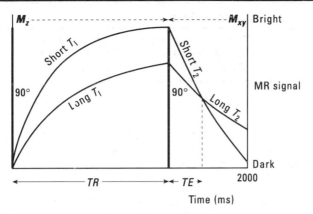

Fig. 8.11 Contrast: combined effects of T_1 and T_2.

Table 8.3 Factors affecting MR signal and contrast

Fixed parameters	Machine settings	Tissue characteristics
Gyromagnetic ratio of nucleus	TR TE	T_1 T_2 PD
Static magnetic field	TI (see Section 8.6) Tip angle (see Section 8.6)	Flow (see Section 8.7) Contrast medium (see Section 8.10)

Slice selection: Z-gradient field

Like CT, an MR image is made up of a series of parallel slices which are imaged in turn. Figure 8.12 represents a sagittal section through the patient with a transverse slice (shaded).

Simultaneously with the 90° RF pulse, DC is sent for a short while through a pair of 'gradient coils' (ZZ in Fig. 8.2), which are additional to the main coil. This current produces a gradient, along the Z-axis, in the static magnetic field. B is diminished at (say) the head end and augmented at the toe end (Fig. 8.12) while remaining the same at the 'isocenter. It varies from head to toe with a constant gradient (a few milliteslas per meter).

Accordingly, protons at the head end precess more slowly and those at the foot do so faster than those in the middle. There is therefore a corresponding gradient, in the Z-direction, of the resonant frequency of the protons. The protons in a selected slice are all precessing with a narrow range of frequencies.

The RF transmitter is tuned to generate a RF pulse which contains a small range of frequencies ('a narrow bandwidth'). Only protons in a certain thin slice of the patient will be excited by it. Only those protons will

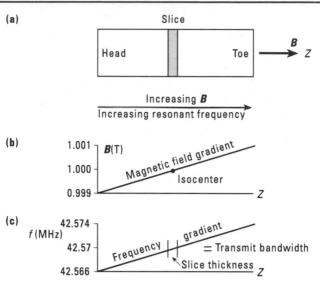

Fig. 8.12 Transverse slice selection with a Z-field gradient. (a) Saggitae cross-section of the patient, (b) magnetic field gradient, and (c) transmit frequency gradient.

tip and, in due course, produce a MR signal. Note that (as indicated in Fig. 8.6b) the slice select or Z-axis gradient field is switched on during the application of the RF pulse.

Slice thickness. The slice thickness may be reduced by either (a) increasing the gradient of the magnetic field or (b) decreasing the RF (or 'transmit') bandwidth. A thinner slice produces better anatomical detail, the 'partial volume effect' being less. Different slices are selected in turn by altering the central frequency of the RF pulse.

A typical slice thickness is 2–10 mm. The RF pulse inevitably contains a certain amount of electromagnetic energy of frequencies slightly higher or lower than the intended bandwith, thus mildly exciting tissues either side of the desired slice. To prevent this 'cross-talk' affecting the image slice, a gap (say 10% of the slice thickness) may be left between slices. This is not always necessary (see Section 8.8).

The slice is subdivided into a matrix of say 256×256 voxels, and the image is displayed as a similar matrix of pixels. If this covers a field of view (FOV) of say 250×250 mm, the pixel size is 1 mm². (Rectangular matrices (e.g. 256×180), FOVs, and/or pixels are also used.) The pixel size determines the spatial resolution.

To pick out the signal coming from each individual voxel within the slice, two additional field gradients are used in turn.

Line selection: frequency-encoding or X-axis gradient

It is first necessary to identify lines or columns of pixels within the selected slice. Figure 8.13 represents a transverse slice through the patient, divided into such columns of pixels. During the few milliseconds that the MR echo

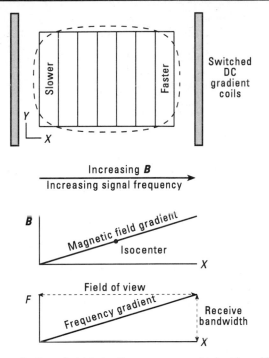

Fig. 8.13 Selection of a line of pixels by 'frequency-encoding' with an X field gradient. (a) Transverse section of the patient, (b) magnetic field gradient, and (c) receive frequency gradient.

signal is being received, DC is passed through a second set of gradient coils (XX in Fig. 8.2). This produces a magnetic field gradient from side to side, in the X-direction.

Protons in each vertical column of voxels experience the same magnetic field, precess with the same frequency, and emit MR signals of the same frequency. But those in the left-hand columns precess more slowly (say) and those on the right precess faster than those in the middle. There is a corresponding frequency gradient from left to right in the MR signals emitted. This is comparable to the frequency gradient along the keyboard of a piano: the pitch of the note reveals (or 'codes for') the position of the key which was struck.

The MR signal produced by exciting the slice therefore consists of a spectrum of RF frequencies either side of the frequency of the applied pulse. The complex MR signal is sampled and analyzed into 256 or 512 component frequencies by a computer using a mathematical process called a Fourier transform. (This is comparable to the way in which the human ear can 'pick out' individual instruments from an orchestra.) This process gives the signal strength to be ascribed to each RF and so to each of 256 or 512 columns of pixels.

Note that (as indicated in Fig. 8.6b) the line select or 'read out' gradient is switched on for a few milliseconds during the measurement of the MR echo signal.

Field of view. The receiver is tuned to accept only a certain range of frequencies, called the receive bandwidth, coming from a corresponding FOV. The FOV may be increased by either making the field gradient less steep or increasing the receive bandwidth. The pixel width equals the FOV divided by the number of components into which the frequency spectrum has been sampled. For example, with a gradient of 15 mT m^{-1}, a bandwidth of 15 kHz produces a FOV of 25 cm. Sampling the signal 256 times takes about 15 ms and yields pixels 1 mm across.

Averaging. The foregoing 90° and 180° sequence is repeated up to eight times, and the signals averaged to reduce noise (see Section 8.7). Four repetitions ('excitations') will improve the signal-to-noise ratio by a factor $\sqrt{4} = 2$.

Point selection: phase-encoding or Y-axis gradient

It is now necessary to select 256 or 512 individual pixels along each selected line or column in the selected image plane. Figure 8.14 depicts the individual pixels in just one of the columns in Fig. 8.13.

Immediately after the protons in the slice have been excited by the 90° pulse, but before they are inverted by the 180° pulse, DC is passed for a few milliseconds through a third set of gradient coils (YY in Fig. 8.2). This produces a magnetic field gradient from the front to the back of the patient, in the Y-direction.

For that brief period of time, some of the precessing dipoles and M_{xy} vectors speed up and some slow down. Those in voxels near the top of the column precess more slowly (say) and lag behind, while those near the bottom precess faster and get ahead, compared with those in the middle.

When the gradient pulse is over, they all precess again at the same rate, and they again all emit the same frequency signal. However, the *phase differences* (see Section 1.10) remain. Those near the top are still ahead of those near the bottom. There is a phase gradient in the MR signals coming from different pixels along the selected vertical line (Fig. 8.14). These phase differences can be detected electronically.

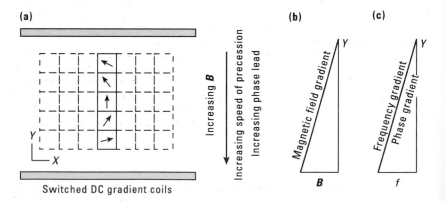

Fig. 8.14 Selection of individual pixels by 'phase encoding' with a Y field gradient. (a) Transverse cross-section of the patient, (b) magnetic field gradient, and (c) phase gradient.

The MR signal emitted by the whole slice therefore comprises a mixture or spectrum of phases as well as of frequencies: the frequencies relating to the X-coordinate of the voxel/pixel and the phases relating to the Y-coordinate. At the same time as the computer is analyzing the spectrum for frequency, it is analyzing it for phase, in order to identify individual voxels/pixels. (A 'two-dimensional Fourier transform' is used.)

In order to map a 256×256 matrix, the whole pulse cycle must be repeated 256 times. Each time, the phase-encoding gradient is increased a little, thus stepping up the phase shifts.

If any tissues move during the 256 repetitions, they will be misregistered, i.e. signals will be attributed to the wrong pixels in the phase-encoding direction. Such motion artefacts, described in Section 8.7, when seen on a MR image make it clear which is the direction of phase encoding *vis-à-vis* frequency encoding. (Similarly, any chemical shift artefacts, described in Section 8.8, reveal the direction of frequency encoding.)

The *FOV* increases if the field gradient is made less steep. The pixel height equals the FOV divided by the number of phase-encoding gradient steps used.

Imaging time. The time needed to acquire an image is found by multiplying (a) the number of signal averages or excitations N_{ex}, (b) the number of phase-encoding steps, and (c) the pulse repetition time TR, and may total several minutes. The overall imaging time may be up to twice as long. Increasing the number of excitations reduces noise at the expense of increased imaging time.

Summary of gradients

The gradient fields are superimposed on the static field. The Z-gradient defines the slice and is applied when the RF pulse is turned on. The X-gradient produces a frequency change, and is applied when the signal is being measured. The Y-gradient produces a phase change, and is applied briefly between the 90° and 180° RF pulses. In practice, the gradient sequences may be more complex than described here.

The gradients are used to control the slice thickness and the FOV. The graphs in Fig. 8.6b show how the field *gradients* vary with time. The steeper the Z-gradient, the thinner the slice. The steeper the frequency and phase-encoding gradients, the smaller the FOV. The steeper a gradient, the greater the power consumed by the gradient coils.

There is a significant difference between phase and frequency encoding. All the spatial information required in the frequency-encoding direction is obtained in 10–20 ms by sampling a single echo; and it takes no longer to sample 512 than 256 times. In the phase-encoding direction, the spatial information is not complete until all 256 gradient steps have been completed, which takes many seconds. This accounts for the appearance of motion artefacts (see Section 8.8).

Multislice techniques

Most of TR is 'wasted': the scanner has to wait up to 2 s before repeating pulses on a given slice. This time can be used to deliver a succession of 90° and 180° RF pulses, each of a different frequency, exciting a series of up to 32 separate slices before repeating the first slice (Fig. 8.15). The shorter

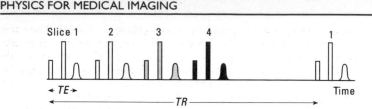

Fig. 8.15 Multislice imaging.

that TE is compared to TR, the more slices can be interleaved in this way. If TR = 1000 ms and TE = 60 ms, in principle 1000/60 = 16, but in practice about 13 slices can be excited.

By acquiring the slices out of sequence, 'cross-talk' (see Section 8.4) and the need for gaps between slices can be avoided.

Multi-echo techniques

This is another way of making use of the long TR. Following each 90° pulse, two or more successive 180° pulses produce successive echoes with increasing TE. Their peak amplitudes decrease with the time constant T_2. The first echo may produce a PD-weighted image while successive echoes produce images which are increasingly T_2 weighted (and increasingly noisy). The sequence can be written as 90, 180, 180, 180, etc. It can also be combined with a one-echo sequence with a short TE and TR, which produces a T_1-weighted image. There may also be time during a single TR to interleave a number of slices.

Fast (or turbo) spin echo

The 90°, 180°, 180°, … sequence can be modified by phase encoding each of the 4–16 echoes (20 ms apart, say) with a different phase-encoding gradient. This reduces by a factor of 4–16 the time (i.e. the number of TR intervals) needed to acquire a complete image (down to a minute or two). However, fewer slices can be interleaved. Fat produces a paradoxically high signal on fast spin echo (FSE) images.

8.5 MAGNETS AND COILS

There are three types of main magnet:

◆ A *permanent magnet* consists of two opposing flat-faced highly magnetized pole pieces fixed to an iron frame. It is large and can weigh some 80 tonnes. It is expensive to buy but the cheapest to run. It requires no power but cannot be shut down and will only give low fields, up to about 0.3 T.

◆ A *resistive electromagnet* is a set of DC coils with copper or aluminum conductors which consume some 50–100 kW of power. The heat produced is removed by cooling water, pumped rapidly through the hollow coils. The magnetic field is limited by heating to 0.5 T. It can be switched off at will, at the end of the day or in an emergency. It then takes 15–30 min to 'ramp up', i.e. re-establish the field. It is the cheapest and smallest, weighing some 2 tonnes.

◆ A *superconducting electromagnet* is a DC solenoid, 1 m in diameter, with conductors made of a rather brittle niobium–titanium alloy in a copper matrix. They are cooled by a 'cryogen': liquid helium at 4 K (–269°C). At this temperature they have negligible resistance, and large (DC) currents can be used without overheating, producing fields up to at least 2.5 T. The machine is correspondingly large and expensive, and weighs some 6 tonnes.

It takes several hours for the coil to cool down and the current to build up. The coil is then short circuited and the power removed. The current continues to flow while using virtually no power. Instead, liquid gases are consumed. If and when the machine is shut down the electromagnetic energy (some 20 kWh) stored within the superconducting coil has to be got rid of carefully.

Vaporization of the expensive liquid helium is reduced by surrounding it with several hundred liters of liquid nitrogen at 77 K –196°C), both being contained in fragile 'cryostats' (vacuum, Dewar, or Thermos vessels) and replenished periodically. Alternatively, a refrigerator system can be used instead of liquid nitrogen to reduce helium losses. Care must be taken when replenishing the cryogens. Air entering the system would solidify like a plug.

The coolant levels must be logged daily. If they fall too low, 'quenching' occurs; the temperature rises, superconductivity is lost, and the stored energy released. If the temperature rises, the liquid gases boil off rapidly and must be vented outside the building. As the superconductivity disappears, the copper matrix takes over the conduction of current.

The magnetic field

The main field must be stable, unaffected by ambient temperature, and uniform to 10 ppm over a large volume. In the case of a permanent magnet, the field is usually aligned vertically, from front to back of the supine patient, while in a solenoid it points horizontally, from head to toe.

The magnetic field lines form closed loops, and crowd together within a solenoid but spread widely outside it as a *fringe field*. This effect is reduced by an iron shroud weighing many tonnes or by additional large coils. The fringe field of a permanent magnet is negligible as it is concentrated within the iron yoke.

Optimum field strength. The static magnetic field should be large enough to produce an adequate signal but not so large that it exceeds the safety guidelines (see Section 8.11). Opinions differ about the optimum field strength for MRI. *In favor of a high field* is a larger MR signal and an improved signal-to-noise ratio. *Against a high field* is an increased T_1, necessitating a longer TR and imaging time, and the greater cost of the magnet. The static field is harder to make uniform, and there is a stronger fringe field, which can affect equipment in adjacent areas. Chemical shift artefacts are increased unless a higher field gradient is used. Motion and susceptibility artefacts are worsened. Potential hazards to the patient, including RF heating, are greater.

Coils

Working inwards from the main magnet coils (see Fig. 8.2) there are:

◆ The *shim coils* carrying DC, which are fine tuned to make the main magnetic field as uniform as possible throughout the imaging volume.

◆ The three sets of *gradient coils*, carrying DC, which are varied to alter the slope of the magnetic field, typically 10 mT m^{-1}. The currents must be switched off rapidly, in 1 ms or less, causing the coils to emit a loud bang.

◆ RF (transmitter/receiver) coils, which are tuned like a radio to the resonant frequency. To maximize the signal the coil should be as close as possible to the part being imaged. The RF coils are of three types:

(a) The standard *body coil* is a permanent part of the scanner. It is used to transmit the RF pulse for all types of scan and to pick up the MR signal when imaging large parts of the body, e.g. the chest and abdomen. The patient should be positioned so that the coil includes the anatomy to be imaged.

(b) The *head* (receiver) *coil* is part of the helmet used in brain scanning.

(c) *Surface* or local (receiver) *coils* are separate coils, designed to be applied as close as possible to the lumbar spine, knee, orbit, etc., before the patient is inserted into the machine. They receive signals effectively from a depth equal to the radius. They allow smaller voxels and give better resolution but have a smaller FOV and less uniformity. They are harder to use and must be positioned carefully. Being closer to the patient than body coils they pick up a larger signal. Having a smaller FOV and limited penetration they pick up less noise, thus improving the signal-to-noise ratio.

8.6 OTHER PULSE SEQUENCES

So far we have considered imaging in the transverse plane using an SE sequence. We now describe briefly some of the many variations that are, less frequently, used.

Inversion recovery (IR)

To accentuate T_1 weighting, an initial 180° pulse is used (Fig. 8.16). This tips the spins antiparallel to the Z-axis and inverts M_z. The spins

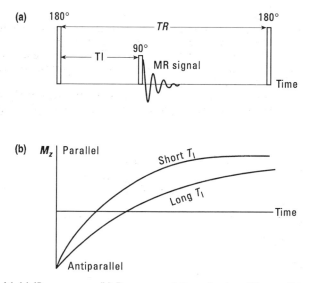

Fig. 8.16 (a) IR sequence. (b) Recovery of tissue having different T_1's.

236

progressively return to parallel, due to spin–lattice relaxation. M_z recovers, passing through zero and reversing direction after a time of 0.69 T_1.

After a variable time (TI is the 'time to inversion', e.g. 500 ms) it is 'interrogated' by a 90° pulse, which tilts the available M_z. The M_{xy} vector so produced rotates in the transverse XY plane, producing an MR signal. A second 180° pulse is then used to develop an echo signal. The whole (180°, 90°, 180°) cycle is repeated. Typical parameters might be TR = 1000 ms and TE = 25 ms.

Consider two tissues of different T_1. If TI = 0.69 × the longer T_1, that tissue gives no signal, as there is no available M_z to convert; whereas the tissue with the shorter T_1 does. The image is T_1 weighted. The longer TI is or the shorter T_1 is, the greater the MR signal produced.

TI is used as a T_1 contrast control. TR is about $3T_1$ to ensure nearly total recovery between pulses. This technique is time-consuming, especially at higher field strengths which make T_1 long, but gives good grey/white matter discrimination. IR sequences can be extended· 180°, 90°, 180°, 180°, ctc.

Short-TI inversion recovery (STIR) sequence: for fat suppression

In SE sequences, the very bright signal produced by fat may obscure contrasts in other tissues. There are several ways of dealing with this. One is to remove the signal from fat by using an IR sequence, with its initial 180° pulse, followed after a short interval by a 90° pulse.

The 180° pulse tips both fat and water protons antiparallel, but they recover more quickly in fat, with its short T_1, than in water. This is shown in Fig. 8.17, which may be compared with Fig. 8.16. After a certain time TI (about 125 ms), half the spins in fat have reverted to parallel, and its $M_z = 0$. Few of the spins in water have so reverted, and it still has some M_z. A 90° pulse at this instant produces a signal from water and other tissues but none from fat.

Gradient (recalled) echo (GRE)

There are several ways of reducing scan times. One method is to reduce TR to 200 ms or even 20 ms. This would give M_z little time to recover and result in rather small signals from the usual 90° RF pulse. Instead, an RF pulse of shorter duration ('smaller tip angle or flip angle') is used, which inverts only a small fraction of the dipoles.

Figure 8.18a (which may be compared with Fig. 8.4) shows how M_z, M_{xy}, and the tip angle θ are related through a right-angled triangle. Figure

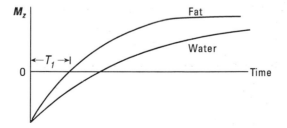

Fig. 8.17 Short TI inversion recovery (STIR) sequence.

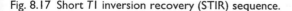

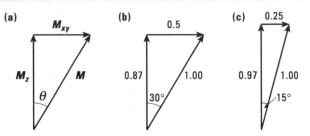

Fig. 8.18 (a) Meaning of tip angle. Relative values of M_z and M_{xy} at tip angles (b) 30° (c) 15°.

8.18b shows that a 30° pulse produces only 50% of the usual M_{xy} and the consequent MR signal. However, it leaves 87% of M_z, which does not take long to recover fully. This ensures a good signal following the next RF pulse. Similarly (Fig. 8.18c) a 15° pulse produces 25% of the usual M_{xy} but leaves 97% of M_z.

With TE typically 15 ms, there is time within the short TR for very few slices to be imaged. If TR is as short as 20 ms the image must be acquired one slice at a time; 15 separate slices can be taken in some 30 s, sufficiently short for a patient to hold his or her breath, but not rapidly enough to produce real-time images.

With such short TE, there is no time for a 180° pulse as used in SE sequences. Instead, rephasing is achieved by a *gradient echo* (Fig. 8.19). As explained below, the gradient field is reversed to refocus the out-of-phase spins. This compensates for the dephasing produced by the change of magnetic field across the pixel produced by the gradient field (see Section 8.3). Unlike SE, however, it does not eliminate the effect of inhomogeneities in the static field, and so the image is $T_2{}^*$ weighted. Nor does it compensate for magnetic susceptibility effects (see Section 8.10).

The usual frequency-encoding gradient pulse X is preceded by a reverse pulse X′ of half the duration. During the first, negative, part of the gradient pulse the dipoles at one side of each pixel are made to precess faster than and get ahead of those at the other. Then the gradient current reverses, and the latter begin to catch up with the former, coming into phase again to produce the echo signal. The peak of the MR signal appears at the middle of the X gradient pulse.

To summarize: compared with the SE sequence, in a GRE sequence the RF pulse is of reduced strength and tips the magnetic vector through a smaller angle than 90°, thus allowing a short TR. The negative gradient pulse X′ dephases the spins, and the positive gradient pulse X, which is twice as long, rephases them.

Tip angle

The stronger the initial RF pulse and the longer its duration, the greater the tip angle. The greater the tip angle, the greater the T_1 weighting (Table 8.4). It is an important characteristic of GRE scans that *moving blood appears bright* (see Section 8.7).

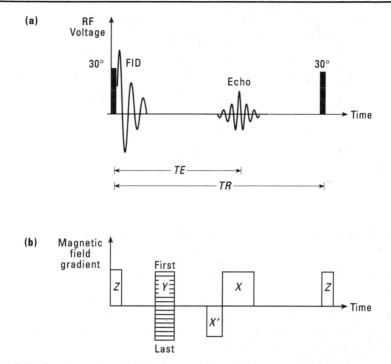

Fig. 8.19 Gradient echo. (a) RF pulses and signal, (b) magnetic field gradients.

Table 8.4 Effect of tip angle

T_1 weighted	TR and TE both short	Tip angle >70°
T_2 weighted	TR and TE both long	Tip angle 5–10°
PD weighted	Short TE and long TR	Tip angle 5–10°

The *optimum tip angle*, which gives the greatest signal, is a balance between leaving sufficient M_z and producing sufficient M_{xy}. The shorter TR is, compared with T_1, the smaller the optimum tip angle:

TR/T_1:	3	1	0.14	0.03
θ:	87°	68°	30°	15°

There are a great number of other pulse sequences, each of which may be known by several alternative acronyms. For example, the *motion artefact suppression technique* (MAST) removes artefacts caused by phase changes resulting from movement, e.g. of blood and CSF. It does so by modifying the field gradients.

Echo planar imaging

A 50 ms 'snapshot' may be produced by an extremely fast form of GRE called echo planar imaging (EPI). Following a standard (90°, 180°) SE sequence and slice selection gradient, the polarity of a frequency-encoding gradient is continually reversed, as fast as possible, each time inducing a gradient echo. The phase-encoding gradient is also switched on and off, briefly, just before each echo, thus encoding each of the echoes with a different phase-encoding gradient. Sixty-four echoes can be collected (in the time $T_2{}^* = 25\text{--}50$ ms) before M_{xy} has decayed too far. In this way a complete 64×64 image is acquired in the 50 ms following a single 90° pulse. Resolution, echo strength, and the signal-to-noise are all low. The technological demands are high. The strong field of a superconducting magnet is essential. Accordingly, chemical shift and susceptibility artefacts may be a problem. Very high gradients and very fast switching are needed. This will induce small, unwanted, currents in nearby metallic structures, and these may cause blurring and artefacts in the image. They can be reduced by active shielding of the gradient coils. Other initial RF sequences can be used.

Imaging in other planes

Any desired image plane can be selected without moving the patient.

To image in the coronal plane use the Y-gradient for slice selecting, and the other two for frequency and phase-encoding. To image in the sagittal plane use the X-gradient for slice selecting, and the other two for frequency and phase-encoding. To image in the coronal oblique plane, apply slice selection to the X- and Y-gradients simultaneously.

Generally speaking, the phase-encoding gradient is best applied along the shorter dimension of the patient's anatomy.

Three-dimensional Fourier imaging

This is an alternative method of spatial encoding. A shallow Z-gradient is used to select a thick slice, thick enough to include the whole volume to be imaged. As usual, frequency encoding is used along one axis, but phase encoding is used along both of the others. The data-processing requirements are increased accordingly. So is the scan time, but this may be mitigated by using GRE with a short TE. A three dimensional Fourier transform is used to decode the information. Usually the X- and Y-axes are used for phase encoding. This avoids motion artefacts in the Z-direction, where they would matter most – especially important when imaging the lungs. The three-dimensional data can be 'reformatted' to produce images of a series of very thin contiguous slices in any orientation, with no cross-talk.

8.7 CHARACTERISTICS OF THE MAGNETIC RESONANCE IMAGE

Spatial resolution

Spatial resolution depends upon the pixel size, which in turn depends upon the matrix and the FOV chosen. A representative value would be 1 mm, corresponding to 0.5 lp mm^{-1}. Using a larger matrix, reducing the FOV and using a local coil reduces the pixel size and improves resolution. Using a thinner slice also improves resolution, on account of the partial volume effect. Three-dimensional data acquisition, described above, has high resolution but a poor signal-to-noise ratio.

Contrast

Contrast was discussed in Section 8.3.

Noise

Noise is a random variation in the MR signal due to:

◆ *Machine factors.* Noise consists, in part, of electronic noise: statistical fluctuations in the numbers of electrons in the currents flowing in the electronic circuits.

◆ *Patient factors.* Noise is principally due to the presence of the patient. Random thermal movement of the hydrogen atoms in the tissues induces in the receiver coils currents having a wide range of RFs, called 'white noise'.

Such noise reduces and obscures contrasts between tissues. It appears worst in the areas of low PD and low signal. The signal-to-noise ratio can be improved by any of the following measures:

◆ *Increasing the signal by*:
  (a) increasing voxel size by increasing the FOV or slice thickness or decreasing the number of phase-encoding steps, although at the expense of spatial resolution;
  (b) decreasing TE; or
  (c) increasing TR or the tip angle.

SE sequences generally give a bigger signal than gradient echo. The signal strength would also be increased by using a machine with a higher field strength.

◆ *Reducing the noise* by:
  (a) increasing N_{ex} (the number of excitations);
  (b) reducing the bandwidth of the receiver so that it picks up less of the spectrum of noise frequencies, although unfortunately this increases the chemical shift and motion artefacts, described below;
  (c) reducing cross-talk by larger gaps between slices;
  (d) reducing the volume of tissue from which noise is picked up by using well-positioned surface coils of good design.

Three-dimensional imaging can give a better signal-to-noise ratio than two-dimensional multislice imaging but at the expense of greatly increased imaging times.

Flowing blood

The effect on the MR image of the flow of blood depends on many factors, including its velocity, flow profile, and direction relative to the slice (it is greatest for flow perpendicular to the slice); as well as the pulse sequence and its parameters. In multislice imaging, the appearance depends on whether the slices are acquired in the same direction as or counter to the flow. A few simple principles can be identified regarding the SE sequence.

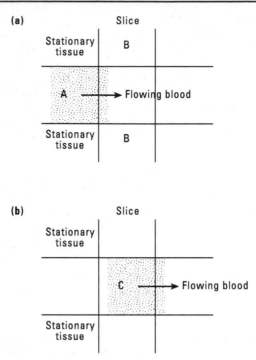

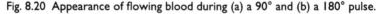

Fig. 8.20 Appearance of flowing blood during (a) a 90° and (b) a 180° pulse.

◆ *Vessels containing slow-flowing blood, e.g. in a vein, may appear bright ('flow enhancement').* Previously unexcited blood (A in Fig. 8.20a) which enters the slice during a 90° pulse is more affected by the pulse and produces a stronger echo than stationary tissue (B) in which M_z has not yet fully recovered from the previous 90° pulse. The effect is most noticeable when the pulses are repeated rapidly, with a short TR.

◆ *Vessels containing fast-flowing blood, e.g. in the aorta, appear dark or void.* Some of the blood (C in Fig. 8.20b) excited by the 90° pulse has already left the slice before the 180° pulse occurs, and so produces no echo signal.

◆ *Turbulent flow produces a rapid loss of coherence, thus reducing M_{xy}, and usually appears dark.*

In a GRE scan, *flowing blood and CSF usually appear bright,* for the following reason. The RF pulses, which are rapidly repeated excite spins only in the selected slice, but the gradient pulse (unlike the 180° pulse in SE) rephases all spins whether in the slice or outside it. Even if (as in the second principle above) some of the excited blood has left the slice, the gradient pulse will rephase it, and it will still produce a signal. Flowing blood does not therefore appear black. On the contrary (as in the first principle above), the inflowing blood will give a larger signal and appear brighter than stationary tissues which have previously been repeatedly excited.

Magnetic resonance angiography

To image only the blood vessels, moving blood is recognized either by (a) its increased brightness on a GRE ('time of flight angiography') or by (b) the phase change caused by movement along the magnetic field gradient ('phase contrast angiography'). Stationary tissue shows no net phase change. No contrast medium is required because of the large difference in the MR signals from flowing blood and tissue. A series of images, stacked in the direction of the vessel, is produced, stored in the computer, and a maximum intensity projection (MIP) (see Section 4.3.4) made onto a single plane.

Chemical shift

The spinning protons are affected to some extent by the magnetic fields of atomic electrons circulating in nearby atoms. The resonant frequency of a proton is therefore affected by its chemical environment. Measurement of this 'chemical shift' can give information about molecular structure.

Fat and water. The valence electrons in the H–O bond in water produce a slightly smaller magnetic field in the region of the proton than do those in the H–C bond in lipids. As a result, the resonant frequency of the proton is about 3 ppm greater in fat than in water.

Chemical shift artefact

The imaging system cannot distinguish whether changes in resonant frequency are due to (a) chemical shift or to (b) the frequency-encoding gradient. Both are interpreted as a displacement *in the frequency-encoding direction*. Compared to water, fat, with its slightly higher resonant frequency, is falsely allocated to locations a few pixels up the gradient. For example, kidney is displaced relative to perinephric fat (Fig. 8.21). A white band is produced where the signal from fat is superimposed on that from water, and a black band where neither produces a signal. Similar effects are seen with fat around the optic nerve and at the margins of vertebral bodies. The stronger the static field of the machine, the greater the shift in

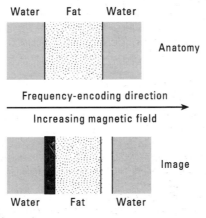

Fig. 8.21 Chemical shift artefact.

terms of pixels. It can be reduced by using (a) a steeper gradient or (b) a wider receiver bandwidth (although the latter lets through more noise).

Chemical shift imaging

The difference in resonant frequencies can be exploited to produce separate images of water and fat. These can then be superimposed with perfect registration between fat and water, thus eliminating chemical shift artefacts. Two methods can be used:

◈ After the 90° pulse in a conventional MR scan, the dipoles in water and fat precess at slightly different rates and are continually going in and out of phase with each other, every few milliseconds. A (water + fat) image is obtained by applying the 180° pulse when they are exactly in phase and a (water − fat) image is obtained by slightly delaying the 180° pulse until they are exactly out of phase. Adding these two images produces a water-only image and subtracting them gives a fat-only image.

◈ Separate images of water and fat can be obtained by tuning the RF system very precisely to the two resonant frequencies in turn. The static field must be very uniform. Frequency encoding cannot be used, and phase-encoding must be employed in both X- and Y-directions, requiring, say, 256×256 separate pulse cycles, and making for a long acquisition time.

8.8 ARTEFACTS

Artefacts are caused by cross-talk (see Section 8.4) and chemical shift (see Section 8.7). Susceptibility artefacts are described in Section 8.10. Other important artefacts include the following.

A *central line* or 'zipper' artefacts is produced across the middle of the image (usually *in the phase-encoding direction*) due to RF leaking from the transmitter to the receiver. Line artefacts can also be produced by RF interference from outside, the patient acting as an aerial, e.g. when the shielded door (see Section 8.11) is ajar.

Implants of *ferrous materials* distort the local magnetic field and can distort or even black out quite a large surrounding area of the image.

Truncation or 'ringing' refers to the parallel striations which can appear at high contrast interfaces, e.g. between fat and muscle, or CSF and the spinal cord. This is similar to the artefact encountered in CT (see Section 4.3) due to insufficiently frequent sampling. This is more likely *in the phase-encoding direction*. It can be reduced by increasing the matrix or reducing the FOV.

Aliasing

Aliasing is a sign that the FOV is too small. It occurs if that part of the patient which is excited by the RF overlaps the chosen FOV. Then signals picked up by the body coil from tissues outside the FOV are falsely allocated to pixels within the matrix. This can produce image wrap-round *in the phase-encoding direction*. Part of the image is shifted bodily to the opposite side from its true anatomy.

The electronic circuits are designed to suppress aliasing in the frequency-encoding direction. Aliasing in the phase-encoding direction can be reduced by:

◆ An 'anti-aliasing' technique, for example: doubling the FOV in the phase-encoding direction and at the same time doubling the number of phase-encoding steps (to keep the same pixel size); halving N_{ex} to keep the same imaging time and signal-to-noise ratio; and displaying only the central half of the image (i.e. covering the original FOV).

◆ Interchanging the frequency and phase-encoding directions.

◆ Using a surface coil which more closely matches the FOV.

Motion artefacts

Patients may find it hard to keep still during the long imaging time. As explained in Section 8.4, frequency encoding happens so quickly and phase encoding so slowly that the effects of motion are usually apparent only *in the phase-encoding direction*. As well as causing blurring or smearing of the image, motion can be responsible for ghost images. Cyclical motion of tissues due to heart motion or breathing can produce multiple images in the phase-encoding direction of, for example, the abdominal aorta or any pulsating vessel.

Cardiac triggering can be used to reduce cardiac motion artefacts. The pulse sequence is triggered by the R-wave and TR made equal to the RR interval. The acquisition of data is thereby synchronized with cardiac motion. Respiratory triggering is also possible but more difficult because the motion is slower. Reliance is usually placed on a fast scan with breath holding.

Pulsatile flow in arteries and the chambers of the heart can also produce multiple ghost images, e.g. of the aorta, in the phase-encoding direction. The faster the motion, the wider the spacing of the ghosts.

8.9 OTHER NUCLIDES

In nuclei other than hydrogen, the protons pair off. Each of the pair spins in opposite directions so that their magnetic effects cancel out. A neutron also has spin and acts as a magnetic dipole, suggesting that it has within it an uneven distribution of equal positive and negative charges. Neutrons too pair off, with the result that nuclei with even numbers of protons and even numbers of neutrons (even Z and even A) cannot show magnetic resonance ($\gamma = 0$). Those with an odd number of protons or an odd number of neutrons can do so. Different nuclides have different gyromagnetic ratios.

For MRI to be feasible a nuclide must have a high gyromagnetic ratio, the isotope must be abundant in the element, and the element must be abundant in the human body. Of the four most abundant elements in the human body, ^1H is, on all three counts, the easiest to image. ^{16}O, ^{14}N, and ^{12}C possess no nuclear magnetism. ^{13}C has an odd number of neutrons but accounts for only 1% of carbon atoms. With a sufficiently strong magnetic field it is possible to image ^{31}P, which has a lower gyromagnetic ratio (17.2 MHz at 1 T) and is several times less abundant than ^1H, but the metabolism of which is of some interest.

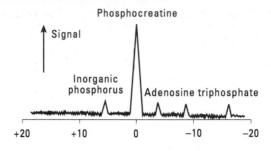

Fig. 8.22 MR spectroscopy.

Magnetic resonance spectroscopic imaging

Because of chemical shift, phosphorus nuclei have different resonant frequencies when bound in inorganic salts, adenosine triphosphate, phospho mono ester, phospho diester and phosphocreatine. Using a broadband RF pulse, all of these can be made to resonate. The MR signals from a defined volume of tissue can be analyzed as a frequency spectrum (Fig. 8.22) and each of the metabolites can be imaged separately. Sequential imaging allows the study of their metabolism *in vivo*.

A high magnetic field (2 T or more) necessitates a superconducting magnet to give sufficient signal strength and sufficiently good spectral resolution. It must be uniform to better than 1 ppm. Because spectroscopy depends on frequency, only phase-encoding gradients can be used in imaging. Accordingly, to reduce imaging time, much larger pixels in a coarser matrix of 1 cm pixels must be used.

It is not at present practicable to image with MR other nuclides (such as ^{19}F or ^{13}C) and other metabolites, although they are routinely assessed *in vitro*.

8.10 ATOMIC MAGNETISM

Paramagnetic contrast media

In atoms, as well as orbiting the nucleus, the extranuclear electrons are spinning, and so act as magnetic dipoles, which are actually much stronger than nuclear ones. Mostly they pair off, spinning in opposite directions and effectively cancelling out their magnetic fields. In paramagnetic materials some of the electrons are unpaired, and the atoms have a net magnetism which is 1000 or more times greater than nuclear magnetism. Each such atom can affect a large number of nearby hydrogen nuclei, as described below.

Gadolinium (as the ion Gd^{3+}) is a uniquely suitable material to use as, having seven unpaired electrons, it is strongly paramagnetic. Being very toxic it is chelated with diethylenetriaminepentaacetic acid (DTPA), which is water-soluble, and to which it remains bound until after excretion.

Used as an intravenous contrast medium, Gd-DTPA is not itself visible on the MR image. Tumbling at around the Larmor frequency, the paramagnetic molecules shorten both T_1 and T_2 of the hydrogen nuclei in their vicinity. As the effect on T_1 is greater than on T_2 it is called a 'positive' contrast agent. The area of uptake is made brighter in a T_1-weighted image and darker in a T_2-weighted image. T_1 weighting is therefore generally used. The effect can be seen for about an hour, after which time too much of the contrast medium will have been eliminated.

As Gd-DTPA is water-soluble, it may produce increased contrast between pathological and normal tissue. It does not cross the normal blood–brain barrier, and so is used to reveal breakdown of the barrier. The protons in water are more affected than those in fat. Water may appear equally bright as fat, and fat suppression techniques may have to be used.

The greater the concentration of Gd-DTPA, the shorter the relaxation times. Since T_1 and T_2 shortening have opposite effects, the concentration of Gd-DTPA must not be so great that the T_2 effect cancels out the T_1 effect.

Manganese (as the ion Mn^{3+}) with five unpaired electrons and iron (as the ion Fe^{2+}) with four have also been used as paramagnetic or positive contrast media, but are not in such wide clinical use.

Superparamagnetic contrast media

Minute (30 nm) particles of the iron oxide Fe_3O_4 with an inert coating are too small to be ferromagnetic but, being very easily magnetized, they are referred to as superparamagnetic. So too is dysprosium (as the ion Dy^{3+}) DTPA, with five unpaired electrons. Used as contrast agents they produce local magnetic field gradients which are sufficiently large to shorten T_2^* and T_2. Areas of uptake appear black. They are also called bulk susceptibility or 'negative' contrast agents.

Susceptibility

When an iron core is inserted in a DC solenoid it becomes magnetized and increases the magnetic field. A patient inserted inside a DC solenoid similarly becomes very slightly magnetized. This is an atomic and not a nuclear effect. The patient disturbs the static magnetic field very slightly, especially:

◆ at the interface between tissue (susceptible) and air (not susceptible to magnetization) in lungs, sinuses, etc.;

◆ due to the concentration that may occur, following bleeding, of hemoglobin, which is slightly ferromagnetic due to its iron content.

Such unavoidable inhomogeneities of, typically, 2 ppm in the local magnetic field lead to an increase or a decrease in the MR signal, and are responsible for certain artefacts. They are likely to be more noticeable on GRE than on SE images.

8.11 QUALITY ASSURANCE

As for other imaging modalities, MRI requires a regular quality assurance program. The homogeneity of the magnetic field is crucial, and can be measured directly at different positions within the magnet using a special nuclear magnetic resonance probe or, indirectly, by using imaging test devices. The same general quality assurance factors as for CT need to be considered: contrast, resolution, noise, artefacts and geometric distortion.

Quality assurance tests should include verification of slice thickness, image uniformity, and linearity, signal-to-noise ratio, spatial resolution and contrast (using phantoms), RF pulse parameters, and the video display characteristics. Emergency equipment and safety features regarding the special hazards of MRI should also be part of standard checks.

8.12 HAZARDS

MRI does not involve ionizing radiation. As at present practised, following (in the UK) the National Radiological Protection Board guidelines, the threshold for the following potential hazards do not appear to be exceeded; certainly no acute ill effects have been noted.

Static magnetic field

Voltages might be induced in flowing blood, which could cause depolarization, and, in moving heart muscle, changes may be seen in the electrocardiogram. No untoward effects are expected if fields do not exceed the following guidelines:

2.5 T: body of patients
0.2 T: arms and hands of staff } continuous exposure
0.02 T: whole body of staff

Switching of the gradient magnetic fields

Eddy currents might be induced in any conductors, e.g. nerve fibers, resulting in involuntary muscular contraction, breathing difficulties, and ventricular fibrillation. Particular care should be taken of patients with heart disease. MRI may be contraindicated if the patient has an implanted pacemaker. With very strong fields, flashes of light may be seen on the retina and sensations of taste experienced.

The magnetic fields should not build up too quickly to avoid symptoms associated with electric shocks: no faster than 20 T s^{-1}. In practice, 1–5 T s^{-1} is typical.

There is not thought to be any effect on fetal development but, as a precaution, MRI is usually not carried out during the first trimester of a pregnancy, and pregnant staff may be redeployed.

Radiofrequency fields

Microwave heating may occur, especially at the higher frequencies associated with strong static fields. It is usually compensated by vasodilation. The cornea, with no blood supply, and the testes, with little, may be at risk. Heating of metallic implants may present a problem. Skin and rectal temperature rise may be monitored, and should not exceed 1°C.

The *specific absorption ratio* (SAR) is the RF energy deposited per unit mass of tissue. The mean SAR in the body should not exceed 0.4 W kg^{-1}. The pulsed RF field should not exceed 70 W.

The SAR is greater for large body parts than for small; for high static fields than for low; for a 180° pulse than for a 90° pulse; for SE than for GRE; and for high-conductivity tissues (brain, blood, liver, CSF) than for low-conductivity tissues (fat, bone marrow). There may be some hotspots, and some combination of imaging parameters may not be allowed.

RF may also affect the working of pacemakers, computers, and equipment relying on electron flow in a vacuum such as cathode ray tubes, image intensifiers, photomultipliers, and gamma cameras. Only 'MR-compatible' monitoring equipment should be used in the imaging room, and special care taken over the disposition of leads to minimize induced currents.

Protocols for the operation of the MR machine take account of other potential hazards such as the following.

Mechanical attraction of ferromagnetic objects varies as the square of the magnetic field and the inverse cube of the distance. The fringe field, which can extend for a few meters, may convert scissors and scalpels into projectiles. Aneurysm clips may be displaced or rotated in the tissues when the patient is inserted into the magnet. Nonmagnetic materials should always be used. MRI may be contraindicated if there might be ferrous foreign bodies, especially near the eye. Joint and dental prostheses are firmly fixed and present no problem. Patients should remove hair grips, ear-rings, and, it is said, mascara containing iron oxide.

The *fringe field* can also affect some watches, destroy data on computer disks and credit cards, distort nearby video displays, and affect photomultipliers. It is minimized by the design of the coil and the use of iron shielding. The area around the main magnet must be carefully supervised. On account of the effect on implanted pacemakers, free access of the public is limited to areas where the field is less than 0.5 mT. In case of emergency the magnetic field should be switched off, although this is not really practicable with a superconducting magnet except in the event of fire.

Other factors

The patient may experience claustrophobia or be distressed by the loud percussive noise produced by the repeatedly switching gradient fields, particularly with GRE. Ear plugs should be used. Accidental quenching, releasing helium and nitrogen cooling gases into the room, can affect the patient, might cause suffocation, or produce frostbite. There is a risk from the use of contrast agents.

Siting of the machine

Siting of the machine should take account of:

◆ steel girders and reinforced concrete, which may become magnetized in the fringe field, and moving elevators and vehicles, all of which can distort the main field; and

◆ lifts and power cables, which may cause RF interference and so distort the image and also produce linear artefacts (see Section 8.8).

The walls of the room incorporate wire mesh (a Faraday cage) to screen the imager from such external RF interference. Doors are similarly screened, and also interlocked to ensure that they are properly closed during imaging.

8.13 SUMMARY

Table 8.5 lists the favorable effects of changing each parameter. Note that the favorable effects of increasing a parameter will be also the drawbacks of decreasing it, and vice versa.

Table 8.5 Favorable effects of changing imaging parameters

Increasing TR	*Decreasing TR*
SNR increases	Scan time shortens
Allows more slices	T_1 contrast may increase
Increasing TE	*Decreasing TE*
T_2 contrast may increase	SNR increases
	Allows more slices
Increasing the slice thickness	*Decreasing the slice thickness*
SNR increases	Spatial resolution increases
Larger volume scanned	Partial volume effects lessen
Increasing the slice interspace	*Decreasing the slice interspace*
Larger volume scanned	Less chance of pathology
Cross-talk reduces	escaping detection
Increasing the matrix (smaller pixels)	*Decreasing the matrix (larger pixels)*
Spatial resolution improves	SNR increases
	Scan time shortens
Increasing N_{ex}	*Decreasing N_{ex}*
SNR increases	Scan time shortens
Increasing the FOV	*Reducing the FOV*
Image covers larger area	Spatial resolution improves
SNR improves	
Aliasing artefacts less likely	
Use of a body or head coil	*Use of a local coil*
Gives large FOV	SNR increases
	Motion artefacts less likely
	Aliasing artefacts less likely

SNR, signal-to-noise ratio.

Special features of magnetic resonance imaging

◈ Ionizing radiation is not involved.
◈ Images can be obtained simultaneously in a number of planes, at any angle.
◈ Soft tissue contrast is high. The range of T_1 and T_2 values in soft tissue (see Table 8.1) is even wider than the range of CT numbers (see Fig. 4.16).
◈ Bone and air do not produce artefacts.
◈ It is noninvasive, contrast media being required rarely.

VIVA QUESTIONS

1. What is the principle of MRI?

2. Explain what is meant by the Larmor frequency.

3. Explain the meaning of the terms T_1, T_2, and proton density, and explain their differences.

4. What is meant by the terms (a) main magnetic field, (b) RF pulse, and (c) gradient fields, and why they are needed?

5. Why are different types of sequence needed? What are the differences between spin echo, gradient echo, and STIR?

6. What safety aspects apply specifically to MRI?

7. What are the guidelines for the safe use of magnets in clinical situations?

8. What units are used to describe the static magnetic field and how do the values used relate to the earth's magnetic field?

9. How is MR angiography performed and what is the principle behind it?

10. What are paramagnetic contrast agents, how do they work, and why do they shorten T_1?

11. What other nuclei besides hydrogen can, in principle, be imaged?

12. What is meant by the term 'nuclear magnetic spectroscopy'?

13. Describe some artefacts which can affect an MR image?

A QUASIMATHEMATICAL ADDENDUM

9.1 Fourier analysis
9.2 Sampling
9.3 Modulation transfer function

This chapter expands on some of the ideas underlying imaging in general. Although the subject matter is essentially mathematical, the treatment is nonmathematical and therefore in places approximate.

9.1 FOURIER ANALYSIS

Figure 9.1 shows how a square wave signal A, such as that produced by scanning across a resolution grid (as in Section 4.1.4) can be synthesized by adding to a sine wave B of the same spatial frequency, another sine wave C of three times the frequency but only one-third of the amplitude; then another wave D of five times the frequency but only one-fifth of the amplitude, and so on (odd numbers only). Expressed in another way, a square wave can be analyzed into a spectrum of separate sine wave or 'Fourier' components. Curve E results from adding together the first three components B–D; adding higher and higher frequencies would eventually reproduce the original square wave A.

The signal produced by scanning across a single narrow strip of lead can similarly be analyzed into a spectrum of sine waves, but now the spectrum contains a wider range of frequencies, and the higher frequencies have more amplitude. The narrower the strip, the wider the band of sine wave frequencies involved and the more important the high frequencies. This is what is meant by saying that a fine structure with a sharp edge is 'composed of' or corresponds to high spatial frequencies; whereas a large diffuse structure is composed of or corresponds only to low frequencies. In order clearly to image small, sharp structures the imaging system has to be able to handle high spatial frequencies without loss of signal or contrast. How well it does so is measured by its modulation transfer function, described below in Section 9.3.

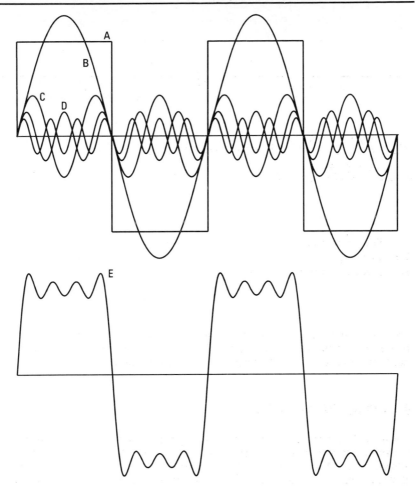

Fig. 9.1 Fourier synthesis of a square wave from a spectrum of sine waves. The square wave A is approximated by E, the sum of the first three component sine waves B, C and D.

Bandwidth

Similarly, the associated electronics have to handle video signals containing high temporal frequencies without undue loss, and they must have a sufficiently wide bandwidth. Figure 9.1 (wave E) shows how the edges of the original square wave are blurred by omitting the higher-frequency components. That is why (see Section 4.1.4) the television (TV) chain in an image intensifier must have a 10 MHz bandwidth when imaging a 4 MHz square wave.

These ideas underly much of imaging. For example, a brief ultrasound pulse is composed of a wide band of frequencies; a longer pulse is composed of a narrow band of frequencies (see Fig. 7.7). In magnetic resonance imaging (MRI) also, a radio frequency (RF) pulse cannot be produced which is both very brief and of very precise frequency.

Spatial filtering

In digital imaging, as described in Section 4.2.2, amplifying the high frequencies more than the low frequencies (by 'high-pass filtering') enhances edges and brings out fine detail. Conversely, attenuating the high frequencies more than the low frequencies (by 'low-pass filtering') has the opposite effect. The same ideas underly the use of 'bone' and 'soft tissue' computed tomography (CT) algorithms (see Section 4.3.3).

Fourier transform

In ultrasound, a Doppler signal consists of superimposed sine waves of different frequencies, corresponding to different blood velocities. The spectrum of such frequencies is derived from the complex waveform by a computer program called the Fourier transform. This is also a spectrum of blood velocities or sonogram (see Section 7.13).

In MRI, the RF echo signal consists of superimposed sine waves of different frequencies and phases, corresponding to different image pixels. This complex waveform is similarly analyzed into its component frequencies and phases by a two-dimensional Fourier transform. This is the basis of spatial encoding (see Section 8.4). Since these calculations are carried out by a computer, the complex signals have first to be digitized by 'sampling'.

9.2 SAMPLING

As we have seen, sampling in various forms is a feature of imaging. A TV image is sampled by the raster of scan lines. A digital image is presented as a matrix of 'samples', i.e. pixels. A video signal is sampled before digitization. If there are too few TV scan lines or if there are too few pixels in the matrix, fine detail will obviously be lost. It is perhaps not so obvious why fine image detail is also lost if too few samples are taken of a video signal.

A complex analog video signal (see Fig. 4.8) is composed of Fourier sine wave components of many frequencies. When it is sampled for digitization some information is inevitably lost. How frequently must the signal be sampled so as not to lose the very high-frequency components carrying information about small structures with sharp edges? The *Nyquist* criterion states that the signal must be sampled *at least twice in every cycle or period*, i.e. the sampling frequency must be at least twice the highest frequency present in the signal. Otherwise, high-frequency signals will erroneously be recorded as low, referred to as *aliasing*. The maximum signal frequency that can be accurately sampled is called the Nyquist frequency, and is equal to half of the sampling frequency.

Undersampling

For example, Fig. 9.2a shows a sine wave (solid curve) which is sampled only four times in three cycles. The samples, shown by the squares, will be interpreted by the imaging system as a wave (dashed curve) of much lower

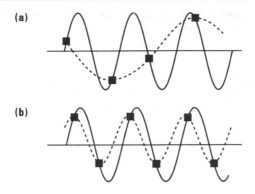

Fig. 9.2 (a) Undersampling of a sine wave. (b) Nyquist criterion applied to sampling.

frequency. Sampling six times, as in Fig. 9.2b, would have preserved the correct frequency.

A stage-coach leaving town in a movie provides an everyday example of aliasing. As the wheels speed up, the spokes appear to rotate more slowly. When the coach has reached a certain speed the spokes appear to be stationary. This happens because in TV the image is sampled only 25 times a second. If one spoke takes exactly 1/25 s to take the place of another, it will not appear to have moved. At higher speeds the spokes appear to rotate backward.

If the phase as well as the frequency needs to be correctly interpreted, the sampling frequency has to be more than twice the highest frequency present.

Aliasing artefacts

Aliasing artefacts caused by such 'undersampling' can take various forms:

◆ In CT, the body section is sampled by a fan beam, containing a limited number of X-ray pencil beams, coming from a limited number of directions. If these are too few, the system does not have the information to reproduce sharp high-contrast boundaries, instead producing the 'low-frequency' streak artefacts described in Section 4.3.3.

◆ In MRI (see Section 8.8), failure to sample the whole of the field of view causes wrap-round: translocation of anatomy from one side of the image to the other.

◆ In pulsed Doppler imaging (see Section 7.13.2) the flow of blood corpuscles is sampled by a series of ultrasound pulses. As with the stage-coach, if these pulses are not repeated sufficiently rapidly, fast flow in one direction will be interpreted as a slower flow in the opposite direction.

◆ A more recondite example of aliasing producing spurious low-frequency detail is Moiré fringes, referred to in Section 2.3.1, and which may also sometimes be seen on digital images.

9.3 MODULATION TRANSFER FUNCTION

We saw in Chapter 4 that an X-ray image may be blurred because of (a) the focal spot size, (b) movement of structures during the exposure, (c) spread of light in the phosphors of intensifying screens and image intensifiers, (d) defects in optical and electron lenses, (e) the line structure of the TV image and the limited bandwidth of the TV electronics, and (f) the pixel structure of digital images. As a result, the final image produced in practice carries less information than the image that would be produced by an ideal or perfect system, i.e. one with a point focal spot, no motion, very thin phosphors, many scan lines, very wide bandwidth, perfect lenses, and a large computer matrix. This loss of information, which is most noticeable in fine structures, is described by the *modulation transfer function* (MTF). Roughly speaking, the MTF measures the ratio:

$$\frac{\text{information in the image}}{\text{information in the object}}$$

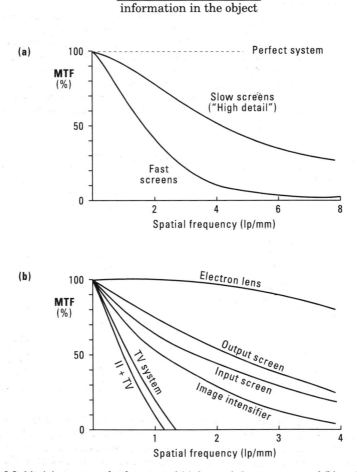

Fig. 9.3 Modulation transfer function of (a) fast and slow screens and (b) an image intensifier–TV system, and its components.

Every imaging system (gamma camera, CT, ultrasound, MRI, etc.) suffers from loss of information and so has an MTF.

One way of measuring the MTF would be to image a number of resolution test grids of greater and greater spatial frequencies, as described in Section 4.1.4. A fine grid of high spatial frequency corresponds to fine structures in the body, whereas a coarse grid of low spatial frequency corresponds to larger structures in the body.

Figure 4.5 showed how blurring causes loss of contrast. Starting with 100% contrast (between lead and Perspex) in the test grid, the image produced has a reduced contrast (i.e. less than 100%). The reduced contrast (so many percent) is called the MTF:

$$\text{MTF} = \frac{\text{contrast in the image produced by the system under test}}{\text{contrast in the image that would be produced by a perfect imaging system}}$$

and depends on the spatial frequency of the object.

With a coarse grid (having very low spatial frequency) blurring does not reduce the contrast, and the MTF is 100% or 1.0. As the grid gets finer (and spatial frequency increases) the MTF decreases. With a very fine grid (having very high spatial frequency) the MTF has fallen to zero, there is no contrast in the image, and the structure cannot be distinguished.

Figure 9.3a plots the MTF against spatial frequency for two film–screen combinations. Fast screens have more blurring than slow screens and lose more contrast, and the MTF curve falls away more quickly than with slow screens.

Table 9.1 Spatial resolution of some typical imaging systems

Imaging method	Spatial resolution (lp mm^{-1})	Computer matrix
Film alone	100	—
High-definition screens	10	—
Fast screens	5	—
Mammography	20	—
Image intensifier photospot, cine	4	—
Fluroscopy with image intensifier–TV	1	—
Digital subtraction	2	512^2
CT	1	512^2
MRI	0.5	256^2
Ultrasound	0.2	512^2
Gamma imaging	0.1	128^2
Computed radiography	5	2048^2

Another way of obtaining the MTF is to image a slit or a line source, as with a gamma camera, described in Section 5.4. The line spread function (see Fig. 5.8) can then be analyzed by Fourier transform to give the MTF curve of the gamma camera. The line spread function and MTF of the focal spot of an X-ray tube can be similarly measured by imaging a narrow slit, 50 μm wide.

The MTF is useful because:

◈ The performance of alternative imaging systems can be compared.
◈ Any deterioration through ageing of the performance of, say, an image intensifier system can be followed, through annual checks.
◈ The MTF of each separate component of an imaging system (e.g. the focal spot of the X-ray tube, image intensifier tube, and TV system) can be measured separately, as in Fig. 9.3b, to see where any improvements can be made. *At each spatial frequency, the MTF of the complete system is simply the product of the MTFs of the separate components.*

For example, at a spatial frequency of 1 lp mm^{-1} the MTF of the input screen of an image intensifier might be 0.6; of the output screen, 0.8; and of the electron lens, 0.99. The limiting factor is obviously the input screen, and the overall MTF of the image intensifier will be $0.6 \times 0.8 \times 0.99 = 0.48$. Adding a TV system with an MTF of 0.2, the overall MTF falls to $0.48 \times 0.2 = 0.1$, the limiting factor now being the TV system. MTFs are sometimes presented on log–log graph paper, in which case Fig. 4.7 shows their general shape.

The 'limiting resolution' of a system is found by seeing how many line pairs per millimeter produces an MTF of (say) 5%. In Fig. 9.3b the limiting resolution of the image intensifier alone is about 4 lp mm^{-1}, but only 1 lp mm^{-1} with a TV system. Representative values for various imaging methods are summarized in Table 9.1. In digital systems (other than gamma imaging and ultrasound), resolution depends principally on the size of the computer matrix.

BIBLIOGRAPHY

General texts

1 T S Curry, L E Dowdry & R C Murray *Christensen's Physics of Diagnostic Radiology* 4th Edn 1992 Lea and Febiger.
2 Jerrold T Bushberg, J Anthony Siebert, Edwin M Leidholdt Jr & John M Boone *The Essential Physics of Medical Imaging* (1994) Williams and Wilkins.
3 A B Wolbarst *Physics of Radiology, International Edition* (1993) Appleton and Lange.

Specific texts

4 Lois E Romans *Introduction to Computed Tomography* (1995) Williams and Wilkins.
5 M N Maisey, K E Britton & B L Gilday *Clinical Nuclear Medicine* 2 Edn (1991) Chapman & Hall.
6 Simone Plaut *Radiation Protection in the X-Ray Department* (1993) Butterworth Heinemann.
7 R Wootton (Ed) *Radiation Protection of Patients* (1993) Cambridge University Press.
8 E J Hall *Radiobiology for the Radiologist* 4th Edn (1994) Lippincott.
9 K Faulkner, A P Jones, A Walker (Eds) *Safety in Diagnostic Radiology* (1995) IPSM Report 72, IPSM, York.
10 K E Goldstone *et al* (Ed.) *Radiation Protection in Nuclear Medicine and Pathology* (1991) IPSM Report 63, IPSM, York.
11 Assurance of Quality in the Diagnostic X-Ray Department 1988 British Institute of Radiology Handbook, BIR, London.
12 Patient Dose Reduction in Diagnostic Radiology (1990) Report by the RCR and NRPB, NRPB, Oxon.
13 Peter Fish *Physics and Instrumentation of Diagnostic Medical Ultrasound* (1990) Wiley.
14 Hylton B Meire & Pat Farrant *Basic Ultrasound* (1995) Wiley.
15 Alfred L Horowitz *MRI Physics for Radiologists: A Visual Approach* 3rd Edn (1994) Springer and Verlag.
16 Peter A Rinck *An Introduction to Magnetic Resonance in Imaging* 3rd Edn (1993) Blackwell Scientific Publications.
17 Catherine Westbrook & Carolyn Kaut *MRI in Practice* (1993) Blackwell Scientific Publications.
18 Allen D Eister *Questions and Answers in Magnetic Resonance Imaging* (1994) Mosby.
19 Making the Best Use of a Department of Clinical Radiology: Guidelines for Doctors 3rd Edn (1995) Royal College of Radiologists.

More advanced texts

20 Stewart C Bushong *Magnetic Resonance Imaging: Physical and Biological Principles* (1995) Mosby.
21 S Webb editor *The Physics of Medical Imaging* (1988) Adam Hilger.
22 Erich Krestel *Imaging Systems for Diagnostics* (1990) Siemens.
23 F A Mettler & A C Upton *Medical Effects of Ionising Radiation* (1995) W B Saunders.

CROSS-REFERENCES FOR VIVA QUESTIONS

Parentheses are used when other chapters are involved.

Chapter 1

Question	Page Numbers
1.	17–22
2.	20–21
3.	2, 19–22
4.	5, 11–17
5.	3, 10, 28–29 (76)
6.	28–31
7.	9–10
8.	10–12
9.	8
10.	23–24
11.	24, 30, 33
12.	5–6

Chapter 2

Question	Page Number
1.	51–54
2.	54–55
3.	38–39
4.	38–41
5.	51–52
6.	52–53
7.	39–43
8.	40, 44–45
9.	48–51
10.	46
11.	47
12.	36–41
13.	34–36
14.	38
15.	38–43
16.	45–46
17.	45
18.	47, 55–56

Chapter 3

Chapter 4

Chapter 5

Chapter 6

Chapter 7

Chapter 8

INDEX

Note – Page numbers in *italic* refer to illustrations and tables; **bold** page numbers indicate a major discussion

ultrasound 188
pulse sequences (MRI)
  echo planar (EPI) 240
  spin echo 223–228, *224, 225*
  gradient echo (GRE) 237–8
  inversion recovery (IR) 236–7
  STIR 237
  turbo spin echo 234
pulse height analyzer (PHA) *125,* 128
pulse height spectrum 126–8, *127*
pulse repetition frequency (PRF) 197
pulsed Doppler 208–9, *211*
pulsed mode transducer 184, *184, 185*
pyrogen testing 139
PZT *see* lead zirconate titanate

Q-factor (ultrasound) 188–90
quality assurance
  computed tomography 113
  digital imaging 88–92
  DSA 100
  films 65, 73
  gamma imaging 131–5
  magnetic resonance imaging (MRI) 247–8
  mammography 77
  tomography 47–8, *48*
  ultrasound imaging 213–14
  X-ray tube 55–6, 73–4
  see also image quality
quality factor
  radiation 155–6
  ultrasound 188–90
quantum mottle 70–1, *70,* 75, 91
quantum sink 93
quenching (MRI) 235

radiation detectors 108–9
radiation exposure
  justification 157, *159*
  reduction methods
    patients 161
    staff 175–6
  sources of 156–7, 174–5
  see also air kerma; exposure; kerma; radiation quantities and units
radiation force balance 214

radiation hazards **148–57**
radiation-induced damage 148
radiation protection **157–81**
  classified and other workers 165–6, *166*
  controlled areas 164–5, *164*
  dose limits *162,* 168–73
  dose reduction to staff and visitors 141–2, 173–7
  legal liability 166–70, *168*
  local rules 165
  medical X-ray equipment 170–1
  organizational arrangements 165
  patient dosimetry 139–41, *140,* 171–3, *172, 173*
  patient overexposures 171
  patient protection regulations 167–71, *169*
  patient records 171
  pregnant patients 158, *160*
  principles 157, *159*
  statutory responsibilities 163–71
  UK legislation 163–4
radiation quantities and units 23–4, 150–1
radiation weighting factors 150, *151,* 155
radioactive decay 119–20, 121–3, *123*
radioactive isotopes 118
radioactive spill 142
radioactive substances, acquisition, storage and safe disposal 141, 142, 167
radioactive waste disposal 142
radioactivity 118–23
radiofrequency (RF) 4, 215, 218–19
  90° pulse 219
  180° pulse 219
radiographic contrast 67
radiographic exposure
  factors 71–3, *72*
  repeated 54
  single 53–4
radiographic mottle 70–71
radiography, children 42, 161, 177
radionuclides 118
  decay 119–23
  desirable properties 135–6
  half-lives 122, *122,* 123
  handling precautions 141–2
  production of 119
  used in imaging 137–8